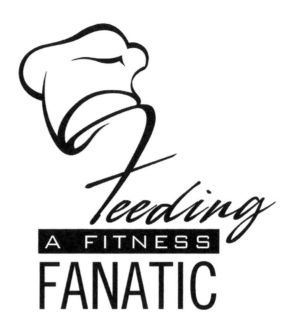

Feeding

A FITNESS

FANATIC

*How to Make Trainer-Approved Meals
While Saving Time and Money*

Elizabeth Van Zandt

With input from Steve Van Zandt

This book is not intended as a substitute for the medical advice of physicians, and the opinions and ideas of the author do not constitute medical, professional, or personal services. Readers should regularly consult a physician in matters relating to their health and particularly with respect to any symptoms that may require diagnosis or medical attention. The author and publisher specifically disclaim all responsibility for any liability, loss, or risk, personal or otherwise, which is incurred as a consequence, directly or indirectly, of the use and application of any of the contents of this book.

Although the author and publisher have made every effort to ensure that the information in this book was correct at press time, the author and publisher do not assume and hereby disclaim any liability to any party for any loss, damage, or disruption caused by errors or omissions, whether such errors or omissions result from negligence, accident, or any other cause.

First Printing, 2013

ISBN: 978-0615815237

Printed in the United States of America

Feeding a Fitness Fanatic
PO Box 1424
Fort Lauderdale, FL 33302
www.feedingafitnessfanatic.com

Cover and book design by Hot House of Design
Recipe photography by Ana Rojas

dedication

This book is dedicated to my father.

Dad, even though you are gone, you will always be the "wind beneath my wings."
I hope I continue to make you proud with the decisions
I make and the path I choose in life.
I will love you and honor you forever.

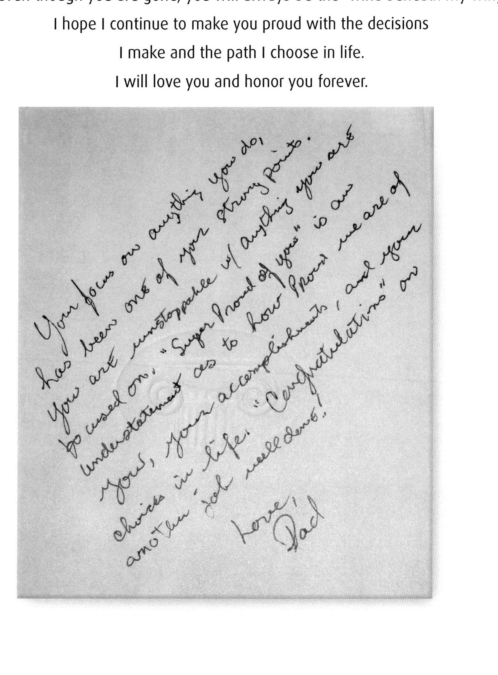

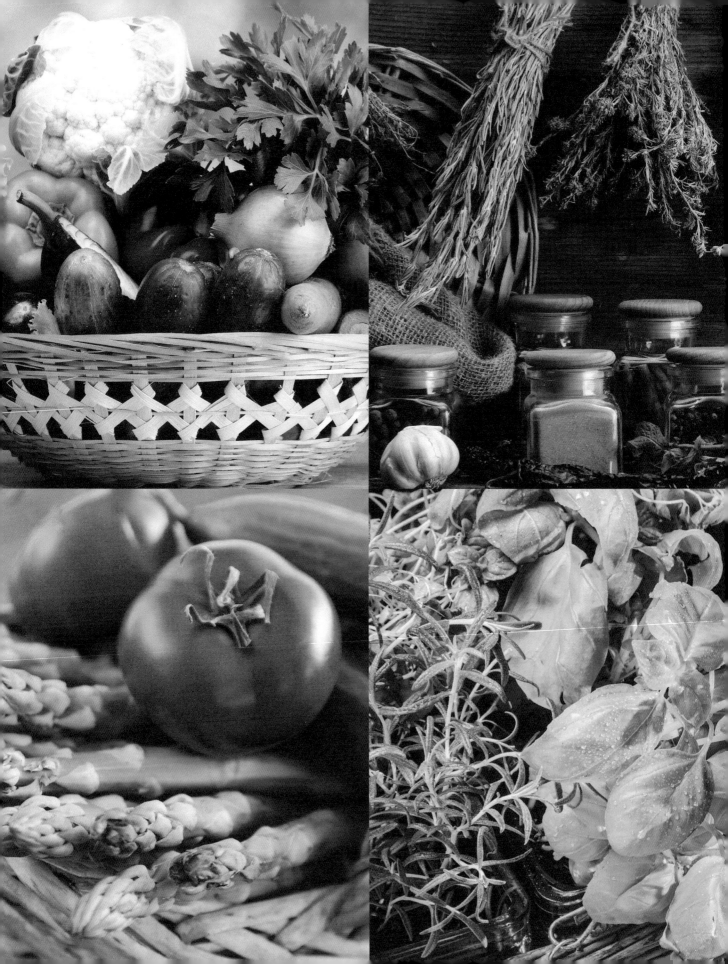

contents

acknowledgments

First I want to thank my husband, who started this all. I thank him for being a technical resource for me and for being my guinea pig (and believe me, there were plenty of disasters!).

To my mother, for always supporting my decisions in life and in this venture, telling me how proud she is of me, and for always reminding me that my father would be proud, too.

To Uncle Harry, who, even with the world on his shoulders, would take the time to actively listen to me and who was always excited to hear what I had to say.

To Aunt Tami, who gives so much of herself to everyone and even in moments of exhaustion, she always showed me she cared and was proud of me.

To Amber, for her continued support and her willingness to try my recipes and recommend them to others.

To Stacy, who always supports me with everything in my life. I thank her for always promoting this venture to anyone she would meet, and, most of all, for showing up and for her willingness to put on a shirt and go to work!

To Marti, for being my cheerleader and for giving me encouragement exactly when I needed it.

To Barbara, for being there every step of the way and for always showing me such genuine interest and excitement at every milestone.

To Terri and Lorain, who always gave me encouraging words despite the physical distance.

To Jessica, for giving me encouragement and valuable feedback, and for giving me insight to what kind of information people are looking for.

To Ana, for always being exactly what I need her to be.

To Cindi and Rob, who both helped bring my vision to life, and did so while having fun!

To Corey, for finishing my title by coming up with the term "Feeding."

To all my fans on Facebook who have provided me with valuable feedback that has been instrumental in the development of this book.

Most importantly, I thank *God*, who has given me the resources, patience, and focus to complete this. And in times of struggle and self-doubt, I thank him for always lifting me up.

introduction

So what is *Feeding a Fitness Fanatic*? My husband is a personal trainer and owns and operates his own fitness company. So for years, I had to deal with all his healthy food requirements. Being a very busy woman (with a demanding job, commitments, and all of life's obligations), I found it to be extremely difficult to balance it all. Cooking healthy was expensive and time consuming, so I had to find a way to make it work because 1) this is my husband's livelihood and 2) this is our health.

So I started really listening to what my husband had to say. His record of transforming clients' lives was hard to ignore. I started doing research—I read a lot of books, watched cooking shows, started experimenting with recipes, and eventually started coming up with my own. I was committed to making meals that did not require so many steps, so many ingredients, and so much cleanup.

I challenged myself by going on temporary eating plans where I could not have grains, dairy, or other common foods that are typically found in many traditional recipes. This enabled me to come up with alternatives.

I started paying attention to the pricing of food and began comparing the various options I had between supermarkets, organic and natural stores, wholesale clubs, Italian markets, farmers markets, online, and more.

I started clipping coupons and researched websites of popular brands I use for additional savings. I researched store policies for coupons, price matching, and more. I asked questions of grocery departments that ultimately provided me with guidance for even more savings.

I tried different cooking techniques aimed at keeping me in the kitchen for the shortest amount of time possible. I started strategically planning my shopping trips to further save time.

After randomly adding different images of food I had made to my personal Facebook page and seeing people actually responding, I realized the interest out there for healthy information. People started telling me to start a blog, but I did not seriously consider it until my father passed away suddenly from a massive heart attack at the age of fifty-four. I later learned that he had heart disease. I was devastated.

At the beginning of 2012, my husband administered a ninety-day fitness challenge. It was during this time period that I really grew to understand where people were struggling. They struggled with affording healthy food, finding the time to make complicated meals, and, on the same side of that, they struggled with tasteless meals.

After contemplating long and hard about doing something with all the information I have gained over the years, I decided to share it with the world by writing a book. Not just a book full of recipes; this would be the book I never had. It would explain why to eat a certain way; it would provide information on the necessary tools, appliances, products, and foods to stock your kitchen with. It would share shopping techniques to save money and time. It would provide techniques to maximize time spent in the kitchen. It would feature healthy ways to make everyday meals and favorites. It would cover everything to truly make living healthy a way of life.

It was then that *Feeding a Fitness Fanatic* was born. It was something that people could understand and grasp easily. The concept of an everyday person having to prepare healthy meals for a fitness fanatic personal trainer was something people felt they could connect with. So, in August 2012, I started a blog and announced the book would be available by mid-2013.

If I am able to help even a handful of people, then I have been successful. I hope that no one ever has to lose someone from a health condition that could have been avoided through diet and exercise.

fundamentals
from the fitness fanatic

My fitness fanatic husband, Steve, owns and operates a fitness training company in South Florida. Steve is one of those who practices what he preaches through the decisions he makes in the kitchen, in the gym, and through his desire to continually learn and grow his knowledge.

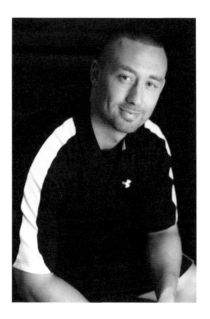

Prior to his career as a trainer, he led soldiers as a sergeant in the US Army. In 2001, he left the military, but took his discipline, determination, and motivation with him and applied them to his passion for the health and fitness industry. After his service to our country, Steve finished college and received his bachelor's degree in exercise science and health promotion. Steve has since worked alongside some of the world's top experts in the fitness industry and has trained numerous elite-level National Football League, National Basketball Association, National Hockey League, and Major League Baseball athletes. Steve maintains a high thirst for knowledge and continues to add top national certifications to his resume and dedicates himself to daily study and research. He is currently pursuing a master's degree in health and fitness management. He is also pursuing a specialty in muscle activation techniques.

His list of credentials include:

- BSE in exercise science and health promotion
- CISSN (certified sports nutritionist)
- NSCA-CSCS (certified strength and conditioning specialist)
- NSCA-CPT (certified personal trainer)
- NASM-CES (corrective exercise specialist)
- NASM-PES (performance enhancement specialist)
- MAT (muscle activation techniques) Jumpstart certified

Now you can see what I am up against! Seriously, though, Steve has taught me a lot and continues to be an incredible resource. During a recent seminar on nutrition, Steve made such an impact on me (and other attendees) that I decided to repeat his message in this book. So I'm going to highlight some of his critical points that should be helpful for you as you embark on this healthy journey.

FOOD PHILOSOPHY

Have you ever heard the phrase from Chinese philosopher Lao Tzu, "Give a man a fish and feed him for a day. Teach a man to fish and feed him for a lifetime."? I can simply give you a ton of recipes without explanation, but if you do not understand why you are eating a certain way, it will likely be difficult to ever change your behavior. By learning and understanding the "why," you are setting yourself up to start making real change.

What is a "food philosophy" anyway? Simply explained, it is the basis of your diet...the "why" and the "how." Most people do not have a food philosophy, and that is often when there is struggle.

Many people subscribe to counting calories, to a low-carb diet, a low-fat diet, and, of course, there are those that go vegetarian or vegan. The fitness fanatic's food philosophy (and subsequently mine) is actually very simple—maintain a healthy digestive system by reducing inflammation, eating clean, nutritious foods, and keeping blood sugar levels stabilized.

A HEALTHY DIGESTIVE SYSTEM

Maintaining a healthy digestive system is critical. Did you know that even if you eat all the right foods, you may not be able to absorb all the nutrients if your gut were inflamed?

How do you know if you have inflammation? What are the symptoms? You may have bloating, dry skin, digestive issues, lethargy, and just plain discomfort.

While inflammation as a response to injury is actually a natural and beneficial process, the United States Department of Agriculture (USDA) states, "Both animal and human studies have shown that obesity is associated with chronic inflammation. Compared to fat tissue from lean people, fat from obese people contains more cells that produce activators of the inflammatory response. In addition, the blood of obese people usually contains more of the different molecules involved in the inflammatory response than blood in lean people. As a result, chronic inflammation is considered a reason that obesity, which affects over 35 percent of the population, is a major risk factor for chronic diseases such as heart disease and diabetes."

What causes your gut to be inflamed? Inflammation can be caused by allergies to foods, by pesticides that are used on foods, and by artificial ingredients added to foods.

According to the United States Food and Drug Administration (FDA), eight foods (of 160 known to cause allergies) account for 90 percent of food allergic reactions and are the food sources from which many other ingredients are derived. These eight foods are:

1. Milk
2. Eggs
3. Fish
4. Shellfish
5. Tree nuts (e.g., almonds, walnuts, pecans)
6. Peanuts
7. Wheat
8. Soybeans

During his seminar, Steve recommended reducing inflammation in your gut by eliminating these most common allergens for a week and then adding each one back to see how your body reacts. He said to drink a minimum of half your body weight in ounces of water (i.e., if you weigh 150 pounds, to drink seventy-five ounces). As he always recommends, avoid processed foods and stick to high-fiber foods like vegetables, beans, nuts, seeds, and whole grains, and increase the consumption of good omega-3 fats. He went through supplements to take and digestive enzymes that can help heal the gut. Most importantly, he recommended taking probiotics to replenish the healthy bacteria.

To maintain a healthy digestive system, Steve recommends continuing many of the steps above even after you've reduced or eliminated inflammation.

Buy "organic," "grass fed," and "wild caught" whenever possible, and eat foods closest to their natural source.

According to the USDA, *organic* "is a labeling term that indicates that the food or other agricultural product has been produced through approved methods that integrate cultural, biological, and mechanical practices that foster cycling of resources, promote ecological balance, and conserve biodiversity. Synthetic fertilizers, sewage sludge, irradiation, and genetic engineering may not be used."

There are a variety of factors to consider when making the decision to go organic. While there is debate on whether or not organic is more nutritious than nonorganic, we like knowing that our food is clean and is free of pesticides and is not genetically modified.

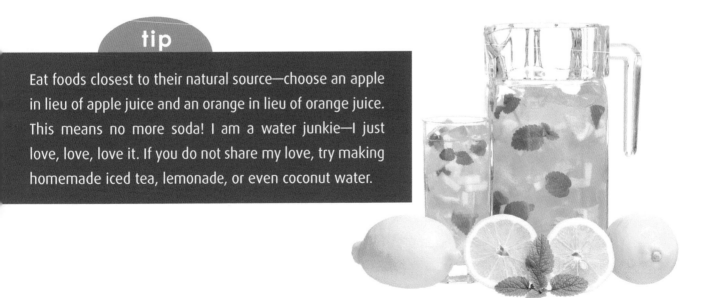

tip

Eat foods closest to their natural source—choose an apple in lieu of apple juice and an orange in lieu of orange juice. This means no more soda! I am a water junkie—I just love, love, love it. If you do not share my love, try making homemade iced tea, lemonade, or even coconut water.

As a guide, the Environmental Working Group (EWG) ranks produce each year based on the amount of pesticides found and label them as the "Dirty Dozen" and "Clean Fifteen." The "dirty" category represents the highest pesticide levels and therefore should be bought organic. The "clean" category represents the lowest pesticide levels. If you do not see a certain produce item on either list, then it falls between the two. Since the EWG only tests produce, I have prepared a list of foods beyond produce, considering the prospect of genetic modification (GMO), pesticide use, and treatment of animals, all factors that can have an impact on our bodies.

While I have not listed organic ingredients exclusively (with the exception of a few) for the recipes in this book, it should be noted that I follow the guideline below and use organic ingredients whenever possible. When in doubt, buy organic if you can.

Foods to Buy Organic:

- **EWG's "Dirty Dozen" Produce***
- **Beef**
- **Chicken**
- **Coffee**
- **Corn**
- **Cornstarch**
- **Dairy**
- **Eggs**
- **Farm-Raised Fish**
- **Pork**
- **Rice**
- **Soybeans**

*For the most current EWG produce guide or to download an app to your phone, go to: *http://www.ewg.org/foodnews/*

According to the USDA, *grass fed* "is the feed source consumed for the lifetime of the animal, with the exception of milk consumed prior to weaning. Animals cannot be fed grain or grain byproducts and must have continuous access to pasture during the growing season. Routine mineral and vitamin supplementation may also be included in the feeding regimen."

Now what does all that really mean? Many people have food allergies (causing chronic inflammation) to grain and grain byproducts. So eating grass-fed meats will help to reduce the chances for inflammation caused by foods.

While the USDA does not have an official definition for *wild-caught* fish, it is simply what it implies—fish caught in the wild. In the world of seafood, this is the term you want to look for. Farm-raised fish is the other option available for seafood. Pay close attention to the farming standards and processes a company is using before you decide to purchase farm-raised fish.

When you start to research what the current USDA or FDA standards are for food labeling, you will be surprised at what you find. Did you know that for a company to claim that it is selling meat, it only has to include 40 percent actual meat in the product? That is just scary, and is another reason why I purchase organic whenever possible.

As part of a healthy diet, Steve recommends eating foods that are high in antioxidants. According to the National Institutes of Health, *antioxidants* are "substances that may protect your cells against the effects of free radicals. Free radicals are molecules produced when your body breaks down food, or by environmental exposures like tobacco smoke and radiation. Free radicals can damage cells, and may play a role in heart disease, cancer, and other diseases."

Antioxidants are found in many foods, including fruits and vegetables, nuts, grains, and some meats, poultry, and fish. Antioxidant-rich foods include leafy greens, berries, avocados, beans, garlic, and more. Many of the recipes listed in this book include these foods.

Stabilizing Blood Sugar—The Glycemic Index

According to the University of Sydney, the *glycemic index* (GI) "is a ranking of carbohydrates on a scale from 0 to 100 according to the extent to which they raise blood sugar levels after eating. Foods with a high GI are those which are rapidly digested and absorbed and result in marked fluctuations in blood sugar levels. Low GI foods, by virtue of their slow digestion and absorption, produce gradual rises in blood sugar and insulin levels, and have proven benefits for health. Low GI diets have been shown to improve both glucose and lipid levels in people with diabetes (type 1 and type 2). They have benefits for weight control because they help control appetite and delay hunger. Low GI diets also reduce insulin levels and insulin resistance. Recent studies from Harvard School of Public Health indicate that the risks of diseases such as type 2 diabetes and coronary heart disease are strongly related to the GI of the overall diet."

During the seminar, Steve drew an illustration of the GI and its impact on blood sugar levels. I have recreated the illustration below. The green line indicates stable sugar levels. The red line indicates drastic spikes and drops in sugar levels, which result in the infamous "sugar crash" we all have experienced.

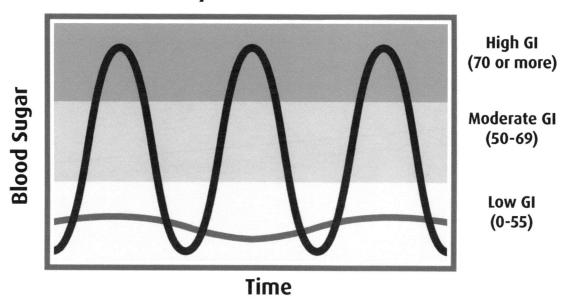

For a searchable food database and corresponding glycemic index rating, go to: *www.glycemicindex.com.*

During the seminar, Steve polled the audience and asked them what their typical breakfast consists of, and many answered with, "cereal, a banana, and orange juice." While that may sound healthy, it is loaded with sugar and carbohydrates with little protein. He explained that a meal like that would resemble the red line path.

What did he recommend instead? He stressed the importance of eating protein with every meal, including snacks. Doing so actually can help stabilize blood sugar levels. He drew another illustration of a plate and showed the proportion that should be dedicated to each food group. It is important to stress that the plate illustration is provided only as a starting point. Your needs may change depending on your fitness goals and corresponding exercise regime.

Plate Guideline

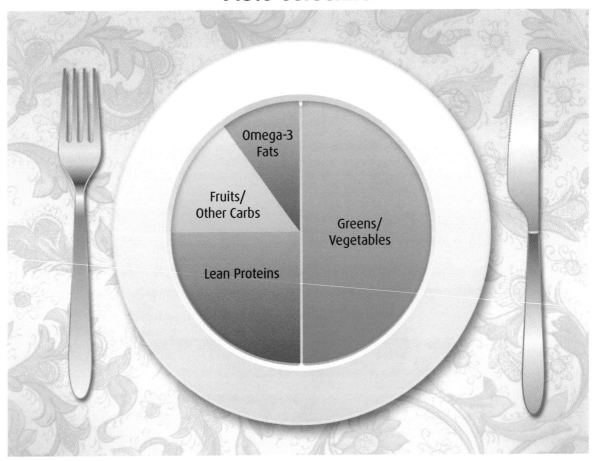

* The portion size for fruit/other carbs is dependent on activity levels. The best source of carbs is low glycemic fruits.

As part of the initial health screening of new clients, Steve always asks about their diet—what they eat during a typical day and how often they eat. The majority of the responses reveal that people only eat about two or three times per day. As part of stabilizing blood sugar levels, it is important to never get to the starvation mode (you know, where you want to punch someone in the face). So, to avoid getting to "that place," Steve recommends eating frequently. You have probably heard that you should eat every three to four hours. This is all depending on your metabolism and your physical activity levels, but is a good starting point. Try eating breakfast, lunch, and dinner and eating a snack between breakfast and lunch and then another one between lunch and dinner. See how you do and adjust accordingly.

On days that I am in the office for a long period of time and do not work out, I will typically eat lighter and reduce my carbohydrate intake. On days where I need more energy because I'm either in the gym, taking dance class, rollerblading (yes, there are those of us that still do that), or completing a long-distance bicycle ride, I will eat more low glycemic carbohydrates. Steve, for instance, is very active and requires a lot more carbs than I do, so his plate will look different.

FOOD GROUPS

Vegetables	Lean Proteins	Fruits	Omega-3 Fats	Other Carbs
Asparagus	Beans	Apples	Almonds	Brown Rice
Beets	Buffalo/Bison	Apricots	Avocados	Oats
Bok Choy	Chicken	Bananas	Chia Seeds	Potatoes
Broccoli	Eggs	Berries	Coconuts	Quinoa
Brussels Sprouts	Fish	Cantaloupe	Extra Virgin Olive Oil	Sprouted Grains
Cabbage	Lamb	Cherries	Flaxseeds	
Carrots	Turkey	Grapefruit	Hazelnuts	
Cauliflower	Venison	Grapes	Macadamia Nuts	
Cucumbers		Kiwi	Pumpkin Seeds	
Eggplant		Mango	Sunflower Seeds	
Green Beans		Melon	Walnuts	
Kale		Nectarines		
Leafy Greens		Papaya		
Mushrooms		Peaches		
Onions		Pears		
Peppers		Pineapple		
Radish		Plums		
Spinach				
Squash				
Tomatoes				
Zucchini				

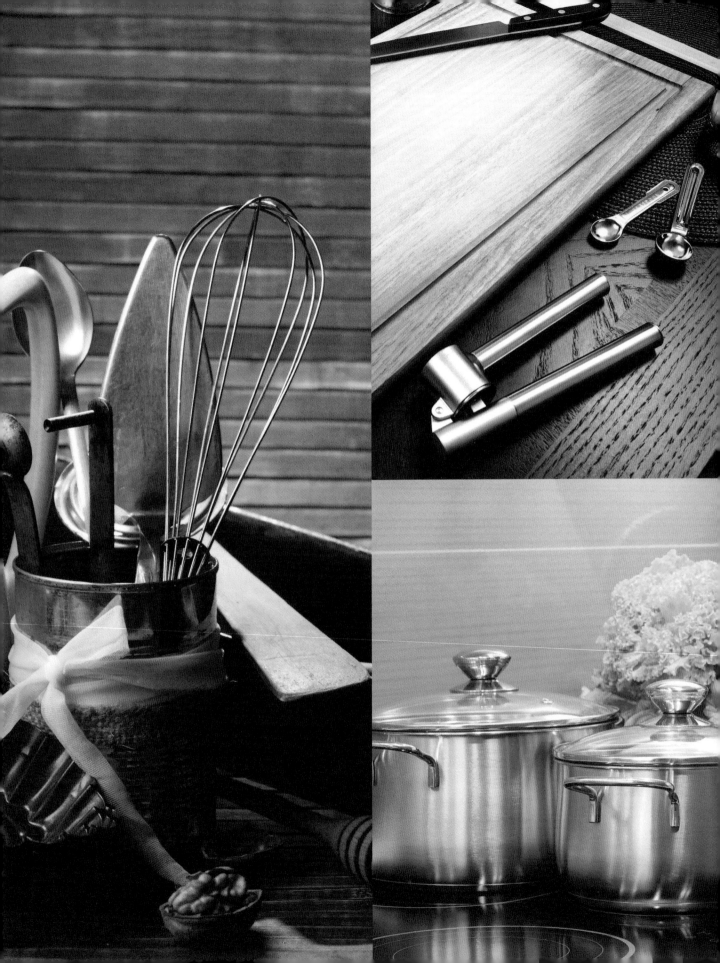

stocking the kitchen

When I was starting out on this healthy journey many years ago, I would have benefited from a list of what I needed in the kitchen, from appliances, tools, and products to food alternatives and healthy staples to always have around. So, since I have all of this now, I am going to share it with you!

Below are a list and explanations of the must-have appliances and tools to create healthy meals. These are affordable, quality tools that can be used by everyone from beginners to professionals. In addition, I have listed some helpful products to keep in the kitchen.

Must-Have Appliances/Tools:

Baking Sheets—I recommend a minimum of two large sheets and one small sheet. I have six different baking sheets, which allows me to prepare multiple meals and ultimately save time.

Big Bowls—Seems trivial, but having several (at least three) large bowls (with pouring spouts preferred) can make all the difference while trying to make multiple meals at one time.

Cookbook Holder or Stand—How many times have you had a cookbook open on the countertop and it suddenly flips closed? After being frustrated, I went searching for a tool that could keep my books open. I found a product at a local bookstore, and it has been great! It works with soft and hard cover books and e-readers, too!

Food Processor—This is an essential tool for healthy cooking. It is a huge time saver for making sauces, chopping veggies, and more!

Glass Baking Dishes—Glass baking dishes are essential in any kitchen to make entrees, vegetables, baked goods, and more.

Glass Measuring Cup and Measurement Set—It is important to have a glass measuring cup for liquid ingredients and a separate cup, tablespoon, and teaspoon set for dry ingredients.

Good Set of Knives—I recently heard a story about someone sawing a sweet potato because her knife was not sharp enough. I felt her pain. Once I learned what a sharp, good set of knives could do, I have not gone back. Some of the benefits include increased speed, ease of cutting, better safety, and time savings!

Hand Mixer—For recipes that call for "whipping," such as mashed potatoes, this is a kitchen essential.

Julienne Cutter—Ever wonder how people can make those perfectly shaped "stick" vegetables? Well, there is a tool for that!

Large Cutting Board—Having a sizable cutting board (like in the cooking shows) makes a major difference by increasing your cutting speed and decreasing your chances of cutting yourself with the knife. It has been one of the most significant changes for me.

Liquefying Blending System *(NutriBullet System®)*—A system that can liquefy vegetables like kale (without little crunchy pieces) has made "drinking my veggies" something that I look forward to! Not all blenders have the ability to liquefy vegetables so do your research.

Muffin Trays—Muffin trays are a must! I recommend different size muffin tins based on the application.

Nonstick Egg Pan—Having a separate nonstick egg pan (without all the chemical coating) will save you much frustration, since stainless steel inevitably will hold on to some of your egg meal.

Oil Mister—While not essential, it is a helpful tool for evenly distributing oils without using too much.

Salad Dressing Shaker—Once you start making your own salad dressing and taste the freshness (and see how simple it is), you will not go back. Any reason to "shake, shake, shake," consider me there!

Single-Serve Blending System *(Ninja®)*—A single-serve blender is very effective for making those afternoon shakes while at work or to drink while on the go. It has minimal mess and is the perfect size.

Slow Cooker *(Crock-Pot®)*—A slow cooker can be a time saver for the busy body in all of us, allowing cooking to be done while at work or while you sleep.

Stainless Steel Pots/Pans—A good set of stainless steel pots and pans is very important. Having the adequate size pot/pan will save you time and mess!

Tupperware for Storage—This is a healthy food essential! Have you ever tried to cook meals ahead of time and then realized you did not have anything to store them in? I have a nice collection of both glass Tupperware and BPA-free* plastic Tupperware.

Vacuum Pack System *(FoodSaver®)*—This is a must-have if you are serious about sustaining a healthy lifestyle. It enables bulk cooking and storage for later use while maintaining freshness!

Veggie Steamer—Whether it is a pot with holes or a separate steaming basket, this is a healthy food must (especially if you do not want to use the microwave).

*BPA is a compound used to make plastic and certain resins that has been controversial because of its possible negative impacts on humans, if ingested.

Must-Have Products:

Disinfecting Wipes—These come in handy all around the house.

Foil and Parchment Paper-in-One—This is one of my favorite products. It has saved me so much time by eliminating cleanup. It is also good for covering frozen foods, such as unpeeled bananas. Due to the concern surrounding aluminum leaching into food when cooked, this is a good option. Put the foil face down, placing the food on the parchment side. You will gain the benefits of aluminum foil without the risk.

Parchment Paper—Parchment paper is a good option for baking by providing easy cleanup.

Plastic Storage Bags—These are good for all-purpose storage and serve as mixing bags for potatoes and other foods to season. I recommend different sizes to allow for the most flexibility.

Sanitary Gloves—I purchased a box of five-hundred-count plastic gloves over five years ago and I still have the same box! Like my mother, I do not like touching raw chicken, so I use these gloves. They come in handy for other applications around the house, too.

Toothpicks—Toothpicks are good for a variety of purposes, including keeping certain foods together and cleaning the debris between the stove and the countertop.

The table below shows the alternatives I use for common ingredients and why I use them. Does this mean I never use ingredients like butter, beef, or white potatoes? Of course not! This table is intended to show you that there are options available if you are searching for alternatives.

ALTERNATIVES TO COMMON INGREDIENTS

Common Ingredient	Alternative Ingredient	Why it's a Good Alternative
Beef (ground)	Ground Bison, Ground Buffalo	Lower calories; lower fat; more nutrients; grass fed, good for grain intolerance
	Ground Turkey	Lower in saturated fat
	Ground Chicken	Lower in saturated fat
Bread (white)	Sprouted Grains Bread	More nutritious; good option for gluten intolerance; low glycemic
Butter (as a sauté agent)	Extra Virgin Olive Oil	Full of healthy fats your body needs
Butter (as a spread)	Coconut Butter	More nutritious; good option for dairy intolerance
Butter or Vegetable Oil (used in baking)	Coconut Oil	More nutritious; good option for dairy intolerance
	Grapeseed Oil (unrefined)	Good option for dairy intolerance; neutral flavor is appealing
	Unsweetened Apple Sauce	Lower in calories and saturated fats
Flour (white)	Almond Flour	Lower in carbs; higher in fiber; more nutritious; good option for gluten intolerance; low glycemic
	Coconut Flour	Higher in fiber and protein; more nutritious; good option for gluten intolerance; low glycemic
	Ground Flaxseed	High in good fats; high in fiber; low in carbs; more nutritious; very versatile

ALTERNATIVES TO COMMON INGREDIENTS

Common Ingredient	Alternative Ingredient	Why it's a Good Alternative
Milk (whole)	Unsweetened Almond Milk	Lower in calories and sugar; lower in saturated fats; more calcium; good option for dairy intolerance
	1% Milk	Lower in calories and fat
Pasta (white)	Spaghetti Squash	Lower in calories and carbs; low glycemic
	Zucchini	Lower in calories and carbs; low glycemic
	Eggplant	Lower in calories and carbs; low glycemic
	Bean Sprouts	Lower in calories and carbs; low glycemic
Peanut Butter	Organic Unsweetened Peanut Butter	Lower sugar; no GMO; pure ingredients
	Unsweetened Almond Butter	Lower sugar; good option for peanut intolerance
	Sunbutter (Sunflower Seeds)	Good option for tree nut intolerance
Rice (white)	Cauliflower	Lower in calories and carbs; low glycemic
	Brown Rice	More fiber and additional nutrients
	Quinoa	Lower in carbs; higher in fiber
Potatoes (white)	Sweet Potatoes	Higher in vitamins and minerals
	Cauliflower	Lower in calories and carbs; low glycemic
Ricotta Cheese	Cottage Cheese	Lower in calories and fat
Sausage (pork)	Chicken Sausage	Lower in calories and fat
	Turkey Sausage	Lower in calories and fat
Sour Cream	Plain Greek Yogurt	Lower in fat; higher in protein
Sugar (white)	Raw Coconut Nectar or Sap (Liquid) or Sugar (Granulated Powder)	More nutritious; low glycemic; great taste
	Raw, Local Honey	More nutritious; helps build immunity to seasonal allergies; sweeter so you use less
	Dates	Higher in fiber; more nutritious
	Stevia	More nutritious; low glycemic

I have been asked what primary foods and spices I have in my kitchen on a constant basis. So, here are my **"food staples"** that you will find are useful in many of the recipes in this book. I buy organic whenever possible. Refer to page 7 for a guide on organic.

Almond Flour (Blanched)—I purchase a five-pound bag online because it is the most economical. It can be stored in the refrigerator for months.

Almond Milk—I use unsweetened almond milk on a daily basis for shakes and as an ingredient in some of my recipes. I buy this by the half gallon—one for home and one for my office. They are usually on sale with coupons, too.

Baking Essentials—Aluminum-free baking soda, pure vanilla extract, and unsweetened applesauce are always needed as ingredients in my baking recipes.

Breadcrumbs—I always have a batch of my *better breadcrumbs* (page 86) to pull out of the refrigerator when needed.

Brown Rice—Brown rice is a weekly menu item in my house. It serves as a stand-alone side and as an integral ingredient in a meal.

Butter—Yes, I have salted butter in the refrigerator to use as a sauté agent. I also stock coconut butter, which serves a similar purpose.

Canned Food—I always have a need for a variety of beans (black, red kidney, pinto, etc.), diced tomatoes, tomato sauce, and pumpkin.

Eggs—Eggs can serve so many purposes, such as being a breakfast, a snack, topping on salad, and an important ingredient in most baking recipes.

Flaxseed—Ground golden flaxseed is used in many of my recipes and is a great addition to shakes.

Fish—I always have wild-caught varieties of fish, such as salmon and mahi mahi, in the freezer, along with a few other fish, depending on availability and pricing. These are at the core of my meal planning for the week.

Fresh Herbs—Cilantro and garlic are always in my refrigerator. I also purchase basil, mint, and parsley on a regular basis.

Fruits and Vegetables—Frozen and fresh fruits and vegetables are used for many applications, including shakes, as a side item, as a snack, as dessert, and as ingredients in my recipes.

Greek Yogurt—This is used in my recipes as an alternative to sour cream (plain) and is also a high-protein snack option with fruit.

Meats and Poultry—Beef, ground buffalo/bison, chicken, and ground turkey are always in my freezer. These are weekly menu items at the core of my meal planning.

Nuts and Seeds—Raw nuts and seeds are always in the house. They are good for snacks, as toppings on a salad, and as ingredients in my recipes. I also always have a nut or seed butter (similar to peanut butter) on hand.

Oils and Vinegars—Extra virgin olive oil, coconut oil, and grapeseed oil are always in my pantry, and I use them on a regular basis, as well as apple cider and balsamic vinegars.

Old-Fashioned Oats—For oatmeal, homemade granola, and as a baking ingredient, this is a must.

Spices and Seasonings—Having a stocked pantry of spices and seasonings will make all the difference. Here are my essentials: all-purpose seasoning, bay leaves, *dry rub or not seasoning* (page 90), fish seasoning, Italian seasoning, taco seasoning, unsweetened cocoa powder, and ground or dried herbs and spices, such as basil, chili, cinnamon, crushed red pepper, cumin, dill, garlic, marjoram, onion, oregano, nutmeg, paprika, parsley, pumpkin, rosemary, sage, thyme, and turmeric.

Sprouted Grains Bread—This is the only bread I have in our house, and it can be found in the freezer, which allows us to take our time using it.

Sweet Potatoes—These are highly nutritious and complement some of my main entrees.

Sweeteners—Raw, local honey and coconut nectar (or sap) are my natural sweeteners of choice used in my baking recipes, dressings, and more.

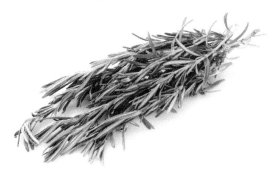

As I list all the necessary tools, appliances, products, and food staples, it is important to think beyond your kitchen at home. As a working professional, I often feel like I am at my office more than my home. So, I stock up my kitchen at work with the necessary foods and tools/appliances to help me live a healthy life. Someone once commented on the various appliances I had at work, assuming the company had purchased them for the employees, and he said, "If only my company would get things like that for the employees at my job, I could eat healthy, too." You know I set that person in place. Remember, you are in control.

In the next section, I will explain the importance of preparation, including how to save money and manage your time to sustain this healthy lifestyle you are embarking on.

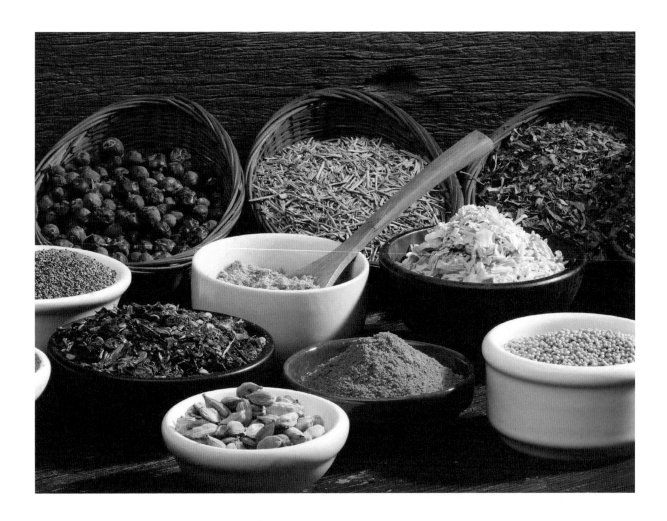

preparation

When it comes to sustaining a healthy diet, preparation truly is the key to success. Preparation has long been a common act for all of us. As youths, we would prepare for a school test by studying and completing assignments. Athletes prepare for competition through physical training and through mental exercises. Job seekers prepare for interviews by doing company research and by answering common interview questions. Politicians prepare for public speaking by doing mock debates. Teachers prepare by creating a curriculum. I think you get the point here. When it comes to sustaining a healthy diet, we forget to prepare and, as a result, find ourselves in desperate situations that ultimately lead to poor eating.

We are all busy, and convenience plays a significant role with our food choices. If you are not prepared, you are more likely to consume foods that are not good for you, because they are often more readily available and come at a lower cost. So how do you combat that? You give yourself options! You have to make time for what matters and it is up to you to determine if your health and the health of your family matters. Mine does.

Part of living a healthy lifestyle is being able to afford it. Learn how I have managed to save money through strategic shopping techniques.

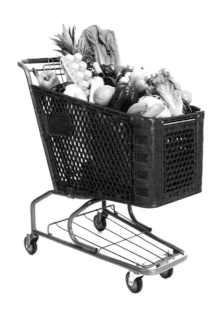

How to Save Money

Let's face it, when it comes to the immediate impact on our wallets, eating healthy is seen as being costly. There are ways to mitigate that, and I am here to show you how. Besides, wouldn't you rather invest in your health now so you decrease your chances of having to invest in it later due to illness? In this section, I will explain how to stretch your dollar.

Strategic shopping is very important to making a healthy lifestyle affordable and manageable. There are many options out there for purchasing quality, affordably priced, healthy foods. You just have to know where to find the deals and how to maximize the transactions. The table below provides a snapshot of where I typically purchase certain foods to give you an idea of where I have found the best pricing on a continuous basis. Do I deviate from this? Absolutely. Foods may not be available or there may be a deal just too good to pass up elsewhere. While this is based on the region I live in, I do think you may be surprised at what stores come in as the best options considering factors like price, quality, quantity, and availability.

BEST OPTIONS TO PURCHASE FOOD

Types of Food	Local Super Markets	Organic Natural Stores	Local Italian Markets	Farmers Markets	Whole Sale Clubs	Online*
Breakfast Meats	X				X	
Condiments & Canned Goods	X	X			X	
Dairy & Dairy Alternatives	X	X			X	
Eggs					X	
Flour Alternatives		X				X
Fresh Fish			X		X	
Fresh Fruits & Vegetables	X	X	X	X	X	
Frozen Fish					X	
Frozen Fruits & Vegetables					X	
Meats (including Poultry)					X	
Nuts & Seeds						X
Nut & Seed Butter		X		X		
Oils		X			X	
Rice & Grains	X				X	
Spices		X			X	
Sweeteners				X	X	X

*There are several online options to buy healthy food much more economically than local options. I frequent Amazon.com, Vitacost.com, and Honeyvillegrain.com sites regularly. Amazon.com offers a prime membership that costs $79/year, but offers free two-day shipping and free movies rentals! Vitacost and Honeyvillegrain offer a flat shipping rate and are always offering discounts and coupons.

As you can see, wholesale clubs really are a great option to maintain a healthy lifestyle. Since they sell items in large quantities, you just have to make sure you can either freeze the unneeded quantity or can use all the food within the "best by" date, because throwing away food does not make you or your wallet very happy.

tip

Looking for a nearby farmers market? There's a site for that! Go to: http://search.ams.usda.gov/farmersmarkets/

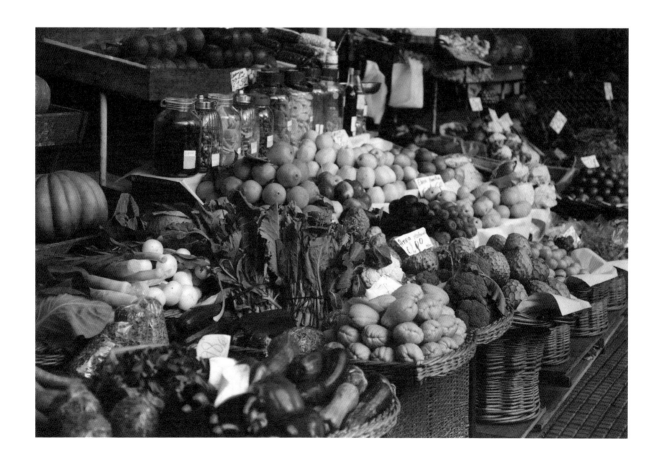

Remember, preparation is key here, so as you begin this new healthy journey, take a few months and go into different stores in your area and find out where your best deals are. You will eventually find a system that works for you.

Now you know that I purposely shop at certain stores to get the best deal based on my needs, but how else do I save money?

I take advantage of weekly sales, store coupons, manufacturer coupons, and competitor sales and coupons. Most food retailers have advertised weekly sales. In addition, they have available coupons that are typically good for a longer period of time. Did you know that on top of sales and store coupons, many stores allow price matching and redemption of manufacturer competitor coupons? This is where it gets sort of exciting (you will see once you start)! As an example, I purchased my favorite frozen breakfast turkey sausage as a buy-one-get-one ("BOGO") free special. On top of that, I had a $1 off manufacturer coupon for every two boxes. I also had a coupon for $10 off a $100 grocery purchase. Are you starting to see the savings here? This is something that happens quite often. Do you know why? Because of preparation!

After hearing from many people who were struggling with the cost of healthier options, I started to outline and blog the weekly food sales, coupons, and other deals for the stores in my region. It has proven to be very helpful for people (including me!). It is my hope that I can expand this list in the future to include additional food stores, and in other regions, too. Until then, you can sign up for the weekly sales ad to be e-mailed to you from all the food stores in your region. How do you think I keep up with all these deals?

I shop at certain places for certain foods, take advantage of advertised sales, and use multiple coupons, but what else?

I stock up on products when it makes sense. If I can freeze it and I can use it in a reasonable time frame, I will likely take advantage of a deal. One shopping trip, I stocked up on so many products that I was overwhelmed at the checkout (even with all my coupons). So, I went home and started crunching my numbers in Excel (yes, I am an Excel nerd) and what I learned was while I may have "overspent" during that one shopping trip, by month's end, I had saved a considerable amount of money by stocking up when the deal was right.

Speaking of stocking up, I went to my local organic grocery store to purchase my favorite brand of organic chicken sausage (which sells out rather quickly because of its popularity), and there was none to be found. So I asked the meat department representative if there were any in the back, and, if so, I would take a minimum of four packages. He came back with an entire case and informed me that I would get a 10 percent discount if I bought the case. I said to myself—it is an extremely hard product to find, I can freeze it and use it in a reasonable time, and I get a discount? It was a no brainer. So, do not be shy. Ask if you can get bulk discounts, and if it makes sense for you, then go for it!

> **tip**
> Just because you may not need a coupon right away, it doesn't mean it won't come in handy in the near future. So clip that coupon! I keep an envelope in my purse or in my vehicle (i.e., I never leave home without it!) so I can always take advantage of a deal.

We have all been there: a product is on sale but there are not any available to buy. I will take a rain check, please! If you are unfamiliar with a rain check, it allows you to take advantage of a sales price past when the item is on sale by virtue of a written voucher. This has actually worked well in my favor several times because I did not need the item at the time, but by getting a rain check, I preserved the sales price for when I did need it.

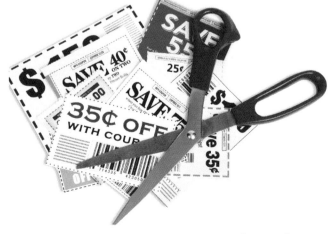

Here is what to do: Take a picture of the product sales sign, and then, after you check out, go to customer service for a rain check. Show the representative the photo (to save him or her time from having to go back to the department to check on the product information) and ask him or her to write down the maximum quantity you are allowed to buy. You do not have to purchase that many, but it provides you with the flexibility to do so if you wish. Keep your rain check in your coupon envelope so you will have it when you need it!

So, I shop strategically, use multiple coupons, stock up, ask for bulk discounts, and use rain checks. There is more!

Many people are not aware that you do not have to buy the pre packaged produce or meat products that are on display. Fresh produce and meats are typically based on weight (per pound), so if, for instance, you do not need all four zucchini squashes, then pierce the plastic and pull out what you need and you will be charged based on the weight. With the meat, you will need to have the meat representative pierce the plastic and prepare the quantity you want, since uncooked meat has different handling standards. This tip will save you money and will decrease the likelihood of wasting food.

> **tip**
>
> Did you know that most deals that specify a quantity for a specific price, such as, "10 for $10" are just marketing strategies to get the consumer to buy more? If you were to buy only one, you would still receive the sale price of $1. So, do not think you need to buy the maximum quantity unless of course it makes sense.

Another important money-saving technique is to enroll in rewards card memberships. Local supermarkets typically have free rewards programs that give you credit for purchasing certain products. I have even seen savings on gasoline from food purchases. The most effective one for me is actually the wholesale club's paid rewards program memberships.

The average annual standard membership of a wholesale club is around $45. While the low-priced products will save you money and pay for the membership and then some, the standard memberships do not have an actual reward component. To take advantage of rewards, you usually have to purchase a higher-level membership, which averages another $45. With this, you start getting a percentage (usually 2 percent) back on all purchases made, and at the end of the year you receive a check for your rewards. Not a store credit, but a check. Some wholesale clubs will refund you the cost of the rewards membership ($45) if you do not end up spending enough money to receive rewards more than the cost of the membership. So, it is a win-win.

My final money-saving technique is to make food purchases (and other purchases) with a rewards credit card that earns points to redeem for hotel stays, gift cards, account credits, and more. This is on top of the rewards membership I mentioned above. Imagine this scenario for a moment:

- You make $250 per month in healthy food purchases from a wholesale club using a rewards membership. This amounts to $3,000 per year.

- At the end of the year, for the holidays, you spend $1,000 on holiday gifts from the wholesale club. This brings the amount of eligible reward spending to $4,000 per year. You then get a check in the mail from your rewards in the amount of $80. This covers almost the cost of both the standard and rewards membership (plus all the savings from the low prices, too).

- In addition to the $4,000 above, you spend an additional $4,800 a year on healthy food and household items at other stores. Using a rewards credit card, you have earned 8,800 points and have enough points for two nights at a hotel for a nice, relaxing get away!

> **tip**
>
> Check those credit card online accounts! I randomly looked at my American Express® account one day and saw a new tab called, "offers for you." I clicked on it and had four offers including a $10 coupon off a $75 purchase at Whole Foods Market®!

Hopefully I have shown you that there are ways to mitigate the cost of buying healthy foods. As a recap, you can:

- **Take advantage of weekly store sales.**
- **Use store coupons (including digital coupons).**
- **Use manufacturer coupons.**
- **Ask for price matching.**
- **Use competitor coupons.**
- **Stock up.**
- **Purchase by the case for bulk discounts.**
- **Reduce those packaged produce and meat products and buy the amount you really need.**
- **Use rain checks.**
- **Invest in rewards memberships.**
- **Invest in a rewards credit card.**

Shopping Time Management

As I get older, I have learned that time is extremely valuable. Have you ever tried to quantify and put a monetary value on your time? I have, and I learned I am way underpaid for all that I do! Life has many obligations, so you have to manage your time to accomplish everything. I have developed quite a time management system because I had to. Hopefully you can use some of my techniques to help you in your life.

Let's start with how to save time while shopping. You probably think I live at the grocery store after looking at the table that lists all the places to shop. Would you believe me if I told you I only go to wholesale clubs once a month? I call this bulk shopping. Who has time (or the desire) to go to big wholesale clubs on a frequent basis? I sure do not! So, I stock up. A significant factor that allows me to bulk buy is owning a separate freezer chest (one of the small ones) that I house in the garage. If you are serious about sustaining a healthy lifestyle, I highly recommending making this worthwhile investment. Not only will it allow you to store uncooked food, it allows for cooked food storage as well (more on that later). The savings in time and in money far exceed the cost of the freezer and the monthly energy costs.

Have you ever tried to go to a wholesale club on a weekend? It is a madhouse! To save time (and aggravation), I plan my trips after work during the week. I do not have these clubs near my house or my work, but I go other places during the course of my week, so I plan ahead. One of the agencies I work closely with and have to travel to for meetings is conveniently located right off a major interstate system. Guess what is between my job and that agency (and subsequently between my home and that agency)? One of the wholesale clubs! So, I plan my meetings at that office to allow me to stop at the wholesale club on my way home.

tip

Pushing around a cart full of a month's worth of food and water can get heavy. So, treat it as your exercise that day. Throw on your running shoes and your workout attire and have fun with it! It sure will get you out of the store faster!

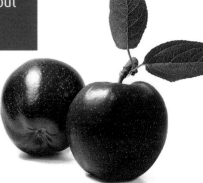

In addition, I am fortunate to have supermarkets and organic/natural stores near where I work. When I can, I will use one of my lunch breaks to expeditiously do my shopping (typically the fresh fruits, vegetables, and other items I did not purchase at the wholesale clubs). I temporarily store them in my office's refrigerator/freezer until I leave for the day. However, if this is not an option for you, then invest in a cooler, purchase some ice, and you are good to go.

What about making shopping lists? Do you think it makes a difference? Absolutely! There are many available options to take advantage of that are aimed at making it easier to shop and ultimately save time. The online account features I spoke about earlier also have shopping list functions. You can browse the weekly sales advertisements online and add sales items to your shopping list. You can also review recipes that allow you to add products to that same shopping list. At the end, you have the option to send it to your smartphone or just print it out. It even lists the aisle the product can be found on! Now that is helpful!

tip

Does your local food store not carry one of your favorite products? Did you know that you could request them to start carrying a specific product? All you have to do is provide the department with the product detail. You know I have!

While I make every effort to make efficient use of my time while shopping, I do enjoy a good farmers' market. Take the time to talk to the exhibitors. You can learn a lot from them.

The long and short of managing your time while shopping is to think ahead and have a plan. It will go a long way with saving you time (and likely money, too).

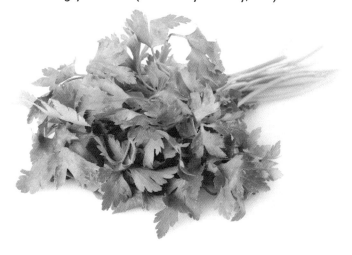

Time Management in the Kitchen

Managing my time in the kitchen has been at the center of this commitment to eating healthy. Once I developed a routine that was comfortable for me, I suddenly was happier, and so was my husband.

For years, I struggled with trying to balance all the obligations in my life. This included making healthy meals for my fitness fanatic husband. I could not sustain cooking every night with a demanding work schedule (oftentimes I have meetings after hours with neighborhood groups), staying healthy through exercise and other physical activity, and seeing family and friends. The constant mess that would be in the kitchen from cooking every night was also a problem. I had to find a solution. So, my husband and I started trying new techniques, which ultimately culminated with what I refer to as *bulk cooking, partial cooking and cutting, and leftover lunches.* These three techniques have allowed me to better balance the priorities in my life.

Bulk cooking is when I will make several meals at once and oftentimes will make extra quantities to freeze for later use. Since I work Monday through Friday, I will use Sunday afternoon to make breakfast and snacks for Monday, Tuesday, and Wednesday, lunch for Monday, Tuesday, and Wednesday, and dinner for Sunday, Monday, and Tuesday. I then use Tuesday night to make breakfast and snacks for Thursday and Friday, lunch for Thursday and Friday, and dinner for Wednesday and Thursday. I do not cook on Friday or Saturday nights. That is my deal with my husband, and he is responsible for either making something on the grill, picking something up, or taking me out on those nights. That's more than fair, right? Not only does this scenario save time from not cooking every night, it saves time from not cleaning up the cooking mess!

Partial cooking is when I will pre make ingredients that I will later use to complete a meal. For example, I may pre cook ground buffalo and brown rice on Sunday to use on Tuesday night for meals I'm preparing for the remainder of the week. Now, certain foods will not last all week in the refrigerator (like Friday's breakfast made on Tuesday night or the ground buffalo made on Sunday for Wednesday dinner and leftovers for Thursday's lunch). So, I pull out my handy FoodSaver® System, vacuum pack it, and throw it in the freezer. On Tuesday, I will pull out the cooked ground buffalo and thaw for use that night. For Friday's breakfast that is already cooked, I will take that out on Thursday and place in the refrigerator to start thawing.

Partial cutting is when I will pre cut vegetables, vacuum seal them, and place them in the freezer for future use. This is especially helpful when I have leftover vegetables I won't be able to use during their peak. As an example, I may stock up on sweet potatoes when they are on sale and then cut them into "fries" and place in separate bags in the freezer and pull each bag out when I need them.

tip

Lay out your food, appliances, and tools before making any meal. This will save time by creating an organized environment. In addition, don't wait for your food to be done before starting to clean up the kitchen. Make the most of your time in the kitchen while you have to be in there so you can reduce your time there when you don't!

Leftover lunches are leftovers from the previous night's dinner. Instead of creating entirely new meals for lunch, I just make a little more of the dinner dish, and then the leftovers serve as the next day's lunch. It is that simple. And no, my husband does not get tired of having leftovers because they are different every day!

Invest in a TV for the kitchen. One of the smartest moves my husband made was the purchase of a combination TV/DVD player for the kitchen. It makes the time fly by. Don't have cable in the kitchen? That's okay! Neither did I for years. I watched cooking DVDs, movies, and TV series on DVD.

tip

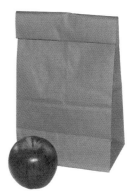

Below is a table that outlines a typical week of trainer-approved meals using bulk cooking, partial cooking, and leftover lunch techniques. As you will see, I make extra food that can be frozen and used the following week. So, there have been times where I had collected enough partially cooked ingredients and bulk leftover meals that I only had to cook one day during the week! It is especially important that I do this when I go out of town for work and want to make sure my fitness fanatic has food while I am gone.

In addition to the meals listed in the table, my fitness fanatic husband also makes himself protein shakes and may have a smaller portion of the leftover lunch as an afternoon snack depending on his activity levels for the day.

WEEK OF MEALS USING TIME SAVING TECHNIQUES

Meals	Day to Cook	Day to Eat	Notes
Shepherd's Cauliflower "Pie" (page 65)	Sunday	Sunday Dinner and Monday Lunch	Make extra ground buffalo and freeze for use the next week.
Organic Chicken Sausages with a Handful of Nuts or Seeds	Pre cooked	Monday, Tuesday, and Friday Breakfasts	I just pull the chicken sausage out the night before since they are pre cooked.
Higher-Protein Blueberry Muffins (page 49)	Sunday	Monday and Tuesday Snacks	Make extra, freeze, and pull them out for use the next week.
Jeff's Cilantro-Lime-Inspired Salmon (page 69) with Organic Brown Rice and Roasted Vegetables (page 38)	Sunday	Monday Dinner and Tuesday Lunch	Make extra brown rice for Tuesday cooking.
Chicken, Baked Sweet Potatoes, and Asparagus (page 36, 39, 35)	Sunday	Tuesday Dinner and Wednesday Lunch	Make extra chicken, freeze, and then take out on Tuesday for cooking.
Vegged-Out "Egg-in-the-Middle" (page 42)	Tuesday	Wednesday and Thursday Breakfast	
Baked Turkey Bacon (page 39) with Fruit	Tuesday	Wednesday and Thursday Snack	
Chicken Fajitas with Mixed Peppers, Onions (page 94) with Guacamole (page 88) over Lettuce	Tuesday	Wednesday Dinner and Thursday Lunch	Use the already cooked chicken made on Sunday and thawed on Tuesday.
Mahi (page 37) with Salsa (page 89) and Half Organic Brown Rice/Half Cauliflower "Rice" (page 78)	Tuesday	Thursday Dinner and Friday Lunch	Use the already cooked organic brown rice from Sunday.

For reference, I prepared a table that shows the maximum time to refrigerate or freeze certain foods, both cooked and uncooked. With as much bulk and partial cooking that I do, it is rare that I have cooked food stay frozen for longer than one month, which is well within the maximum suggested time.

STORAGE CHART FOR MEATS, FISH, AND LEFTOVERS

Food	Refrigerator	Freezer
FRESH		
Beef	3—5 days	6—12 months
Buffalo/Bison		
Chicken	1—2 days	9 months
Fish, Fatty (Salmon, etc.)	1—2 days	2—3 months
Fish, Lean (Cod, Flounder, etc.)	1—2 days	6 months
Lamb	3—5 days	6—9 months
Pork	3—5 days	4—6 months
Turkey	1—2 days	9 months
Veal	3—5 days	4—6 months
LEFTOVERS		
Cooked Meat and Egg Dishes	3—4 days	2—3 months
Cooked Poultry and Fish	3—4 days	4—6 months
Soups, Stews, and Vegetables	3—4 days	2—3 months
Gravy and Meat Broth	1—2 days	2—3 months

Source: FDA

tip

Tired of scrubbing leftover foods off your stainless steel pots and pans? Buy inexpensive white cooking wine or apple cider vinegar and pour onto the surface with the leftover foods while it is still hot. It will start to lift the foods and make it much easier to scrub away. Do not leave the wine or vinegar on for longer than a few minutes.

You have learned the fitness fanatic's food philosophy, what to stock your kitchen with, how to save time and money by shopping strategically, and how to maximize your time in the kitchen, and you have received a week's worth of trainer-approved meals. Now it is time to get in the kitchen and start making healthy meals!

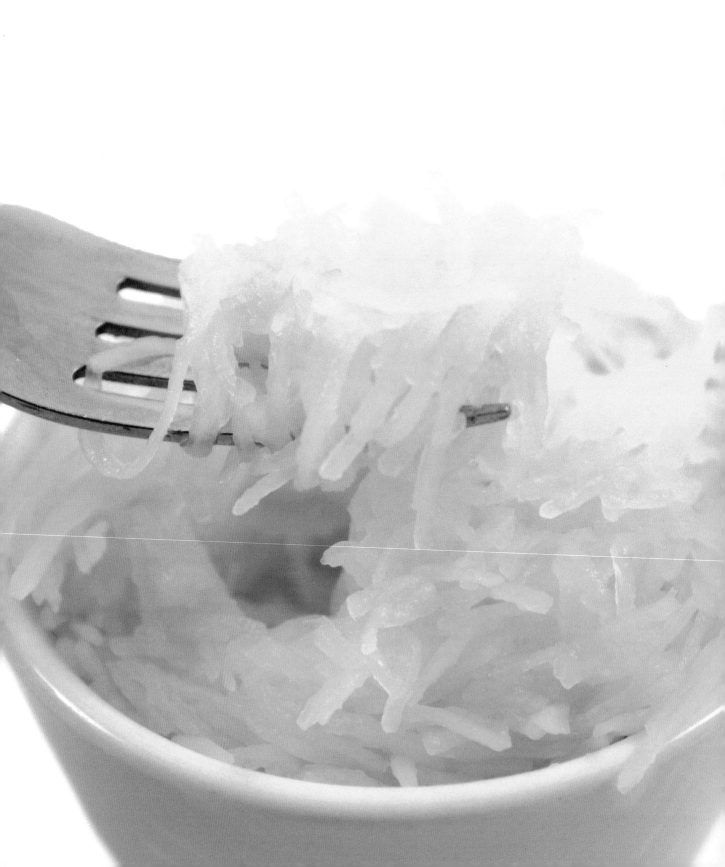

one-ingredient
quick recipes

Oftentimes you just need to make a simple main entree or side item, but you may not know the best way to make it. So, I've included common healthy entrees and sides to complement any meal!

FOOD	METHOD	INSTRUCTIONS
Acorn Squash	Roasted	Preheat the oven to 350 degrees. Cut the acorn squash in half and then scoop out the flesh and seeds. Rub coconut oil on the inside and outside of the squash. Place face down in a glass-baking dish. Roast for approximately 45 minutes. Serve.
Asparagus	Roasted	Preheat the oven to 350 degrees and line a baking sheet with parchment paper and spray with a non-stick spray. Cut about an inch off the bottom of the asparagus, rinse, and dry off. Lay out the asparagus so they are in a single layer. Drizzle with extra virgin olive oil, pure sea salt, and ground black pepper. Place in the oven on the center rack and roast for 10 minutes. Serve.
Brussels Sprouts	Roasted	Preheat the oven to 400 degrees and line a baking sheet with foil and parchment paper-in-one (with the foil facing down so it is not touching the food). Place Brussels sprouts in a large plastic bag, add coconut oil, and sprinkle pure sea salt. Close the bag and massage the Brussels sprouts so they are evenly covered with the oil. Pour onto the baking sheet and place in the oven on the center rack and roast for 35 minutes, shaking the baking sheet halfway through. Once they are lightly blackened, remove, and serve.

FOOD	METHOD	INSTRUCTIONS
Chicken (Breasts)	Baked	Preheat the oven to 350 degrees and line a baking sheet with foil and parchment paper-in-one (with the foil facing down so it is not touching the food). Wash and trim any visible fat from the chicken (making sure you disinfect the area afterwards). Place the chicken in a large plastic bag and drizzle with extra virgin olive oil (EVOO). Close the bag and massage so each breast has EVOO on it. Place the breasts on the baking sheet in a single layer so they are not touching. Sprinkle your favorite seasoning or *dry rub or not seasoning* (page 90) liberally and then place in the oven on the center rack and bake for 35 minutes or until the internal temperature of the chicken is 165 degrees Fahrenheit. Remove and let stand for 5 minutes and then serve. Tips for even better chicken: 1) Marinate in the refrigerator for up to 12 hours. 2) Place a rack on top of the baking sheet and put the chicken directly on the rack. 3) Cover the raw chicken with plastic and then flatten using a hammer like motion.
Eggplant 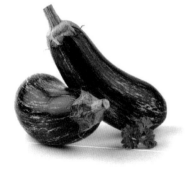	"Sticks"	Preheat the oven to 400 degrees and line a baking sheet with parchment paper and spray with a non-stick spray. Remove the skin of 1 eggplant and then cut into ½ inch-thick "sticks." In a bowl, combine ¾ cup almond flour (blanched), ¼ cup parmesan cheese, ¼ tsp. pure sea salt, ⅛ tsp. ground black pepper, and ⅛ tsp. paprika. In a separate bowl, mix a large egg with 2 tbsp. unsweetened almond milk. Dip the eggplant sticks in the egg mixture and then the flour mixture and place on the baking sheet so the eggplant sticks are not touching. Place on the center rack and bake for 18 minutes or until golden brown and crispy. Serve.
Eggs	Hard Boiled (Easy to Peel)	Place eggs in a pot in a single layer and cover with 1 inch of water. Heat a burner to high heat and bring to a boil. Remove the pot from the burner, cover, and let stand for 10 minutes. While the eggs are covered, fill a large bowl with cold water and ice. Gently shake the pot full of eggs so they start to crack and then pour the hot water out. Transfer the eggs to the bowl full of iced water. Let sit for 5 minutes and then peel and serve.

FOOD	METHOD	INSTRUCTIONS
Fish (White)	Roasted	Preheat the oven to 425 degrees and line a baking sheet with foil and parchment paper-in-one (with the foil facing down so that it is not touching the food). Arrange the fish on the baking sheet so they are not touching. Liberally cover each fish fillet with a fish seasoning such as Chef Paul Prudhomme's® Blackened Redfish Magic and add ½ tbsp. salted butter on each fillet. Bake for 15-20 minutes or until the fish is no longer pink in the center. Serve. *As an alternative, you can place fish on the baking sheet liner and add a ½ tbsp. of salted butter on each fish fillet and sprinkle with salt, pepper, and garlic powder and then fold the liner so it creates a steaming environment for the fish (I typically do this for salmon).*
Fish (White)	Sautéed	Heat a large skillet to medium and add enough extra virgin olive oil so that it evenly coats the bottom of the skillet (approx. 1-2 tbsp.). Liberally cover each fish fillet with a fish seasoning such as Chef Paul Prudhomme's® Blackened Redfish Magic. Place in the heated skillet and cook about 10 minutes, flipping halfway through until the fish is no longer pink in the center. Serve.
Fish (Salmon)	Grilled	Heat up a grill. Brush a marinade onto each fish fillet. Place the fish directly on the grill racks (with the skin side up) and grill for approximately 12 minutes, flipping halfway through. Serve.
Green Beans	Roasted	Preheat the oven to 400 degrees. Clean the green beans, pat dry, and cut the ends off. Place the green beans into a glass-baking dish. Add your favorite organic pasta sauce so that all green beans are covered. Place in the oven on the center rack and bake for 15-20 minutes. Serve.
Kale	Chips	Preheat the oven to 350 degrees and line a baking sheet with parchment paper and spray with a non-stick spray. Clean the kale and then dry with a paper towel. Lay the kale on the baking sheet in a single layer and drizzle with extra virgin olive oil, pure sea salt, and pepper. Bake for 12-14 minutes (watch closely, as it can burn quickly). Serve.

FOOD	METHOD	INSTRUCTIONS
Mixed Vegetables	Roasted	Preheat the oven to 400 degrees and line a baking sheet with foil and parchment paper-in-one (with the foil facing down so it is not touching the food). Place your favorite root vegetables (cut up in chunks) in a large plastic storage bag, drizzle with coconut oil, and sprinkle pure sea salt and ground black pepper. Close the bag and massage the vegetables so they are evenly covered with oil. Pour onto the baking sheet and place in the oven on the center rack and roast for 40 minutes or until they are tender.
Mushrooms	Sautéed	Heat a skillet to medium and add enough extra virgin olive oil so that it evenly coats the bottom of the skillet (approx. 1-2 tbsp. depending on the size of your skillet). Add sliced mushrooms to the skillet and add pure sea salt and ground black pepper to taste. Using a wooden spoon, move the mushrooms around until they are darkened and tender. Serve.
Spaghetti Squash (Pictured on Pg 34)	"Noodles"	Preheat the oven to 375 degrees. Cut a spaghetti squash in half lengthwise and then scoop out the flesh and seeds. Put the squash face down in a large glass-baking dish. Pour ½ cup of water into the dish. Place in the oven on the center rack and bake for 30-35 minutes. Remove and turn the squash over (be careful, it will be very hot). Let cool for 5-10 minutes and then take a large fork and run the fork from top to bottom, removing strands and resembling pasta. Add pure sea salt and ground black pepper to taste. Serve.
Spinach	Sautéed	Heat a skillet to medium and add enough extra virgin olive oil so that it evenly coats the bottom of the skillet (approx. 1-2 tbsp. depending on the size of your skillet). Add spinach (fresh or thawed), fresh garlic, pure sea salt, and ground pepper. Using a wooden spoon, move the spinach around until it starts to wilt. Serve.

FOOD	METHOD	INSTRUCTIONS
Sweet Potato	Baked	Preheat the oven to 400 degrees and line a baking sheet with parchment paper. Scrub potatoes, dry off, and then poke about 6 small holes in each of the sweet potatoes. Place all potatoes in a large plastic storage bag, add coconut oil, and sprinkle pure sea salt. Close the bag and massage potatoes so each potato is covered with oil. Put the potatoes on the baking sheet and place in the oven on the center rack. Bake for 50 minutes to an hour based on the size of the potatoes. Serve and make sure to eat the skins, too!
Sweet Potato	Baked Fries	Preheat the oven to 425 degrees. Scrub potatoes, dry off, and cut into ½-inch-thick "fries." Place all potatoes in a large plastic storage bag, add coconut oil, and sprinkle pure sea salt. Close the bag and massage the potatoes so they are evenly covered with oil. Transfer onto a baking sheet and arrange in one layer so they are not touching. Roast for 1 hour, flipping the potatoes with a metal spatula halfway through. Remove, sprinkle with ground black pepper and paprika, and serve.
Turkey Bacon	Baked	Preheat the oven to 400 degrees and line a baking sheet with foil and parchment paper-in-one (with the foil facing down so it is not touching the food). Lay the turkey bacon in a single layer on the baking sheet. Place in the oven on the center rack and bake for 20-25 minutes until crispy. Serve.
Zucchini	"Noodles"	Remove the skin of 2 zucchinis. Using a julienne cutter, cut the zucchini into "noodles." Heat a large skillet to medium and add enough extra virgin olive oil so that it evenly coats the bottom of the skillet (approx. 1-2 tbsp.). Add the zucchini, pure sea salt, and ground black pepper. Cook until the zucchini becomes tender and resembles pasta. Serve.

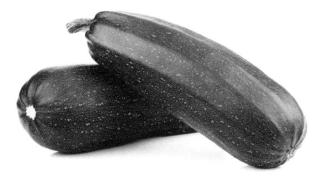

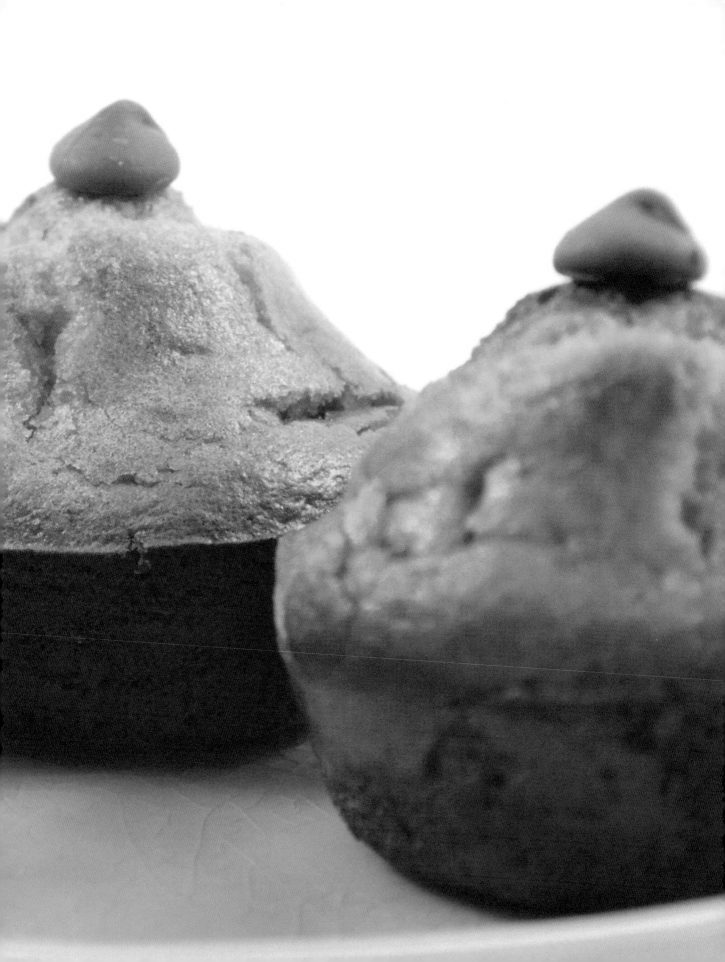

breakfast/
snacks

Vegged-Out "Egg-in-the-Middle"

As a child growing up, I used to love "egg-in-the-middles." So, I made them more nutritious by adding veggies and cottage cheese and by removing most of the bread. This is one of my favorite breakfast meals for sure!

- 4 Large Eggs
- 4 Pieces Sprouted Grains Bread, Thawed
- 1 Cup Your Favorite Veggies, Cooked
  (spinach, mushrooms, and red peppers are shown)
- 2 Tbsp. Low-Fat Cottage Cheese
- Salt and Pepper to Taste

Makes 2 servings.

1. Pull out your cooked veggies and mix in a bowl with the eggs and cottage cheese.
2. Remove the interior of the bread leaving only the crust (just before it looks like it will rip apart). Put the removed bread in a plastic storage bag and place in the refrigerator and save to make a future batch of *better breadcrumbs* (page 86).
3. Spray a pan with a non-stick spray and turn the burner on medium.
4. Place the bread in the pan and then pour the egg mixture into each bread hole.
5. Cook on both sides until the eggs are no longer runny.
6. Add salt and pepper and then serve.

Vegged-Out Omelet

Eggs and veggies are such a natural fit so here's an easy omelet recipe that is sure to please!

- 2 Large Eggs
- 2 Large Eggs, Whites Only
- 1 Cup Your Favorite Veggies, Cooked
- ⅓ Cup Low-Fat Cottage Cheese
- 2 Tbsp. Mozzarella Cheese, Shredded
- Salt and Pepper to Taste

Makes 1-2 servings.

1. In a bowl, mix together all ingredients except the mozzarella cheese.
2. Using a medium sized non-stick pan, spray with non-stick spray and heat a burner to medium.
3. Pour the egg mixture into the pan, add salt and pepper, and keep flipping until cooked.
4. Place the omelet on a plate and then sprinkle the mozzarella cheese on top. You are ready to serve.

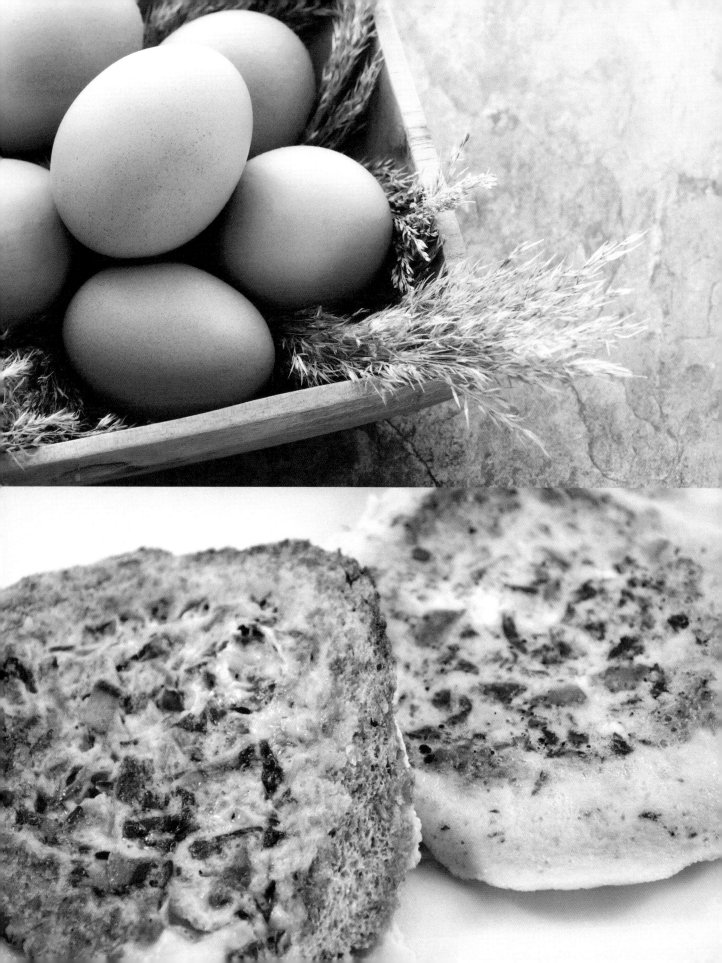

Sprouted Grains Egg Sandwich

Breakfast sandwiches are such a comfort food, but have long had a bad rep. By adding veggies, using alternative meats, and reducing the bread and cheese, you no longer have to feel guilty!

- 1 Sprouted Grains English Muffin
- 2 Large Eggs
- ½ Cup Your Favorite Veggies, Cooked
- 1 Turkey Sausage Patty*
  (No Nitrates or Nitrites Added), Cooked
- ½ Tbsp. Your Favorite Cheese, Shredded

*Alternatively, you can also use 2 slices of *baked turkey bacon* (page 39) or 1 chicken sausage cut in half, lengthwise.

Makes 1 serving.

1. Start by making 2 cuts into the English muffin so that you have a bottom, middle, and a top (sprouted grains English muffins are thicker than traditional English muffins). You want the middle to be the thickest.

2. Place the middle part in a plastic storage bag and put in the refrigerator and save to make a future batch of *better breadcrumbs* (page 86).

3. Put the 2 remaining muffin pieces in a toaster until lightly toasted.

4. In a bowl, mix the eggs with the veggies.

5. Using a small pan, spray with non-stick spray and heat a burner to medium.

6. Pour the egg mixture and cook, flipping halfway through.

7. Once the egg is cooked, fold so that it will fit nicely onto the sandwich.

8. Layer the egg on the bottom part of the toasted muffin then add the turkey sausage patty, then add the cheese and top it off with the other toasted muffin piece.

9. Take a paper plate, flip over, and push down on the sandwich. Hold (or place something heavy enough to weigh it down) for a couple of minutes until the cheese is melted and the sandwich is held together. Alternatively, you can use the microwave to melt the cheese.

10. Cut the sandwich in half and serve.

tip

Have leftover veggies from your dinner date? Save a step and use them in this recipe!

French Toast

Nothing fancy here—just a simple (and good) recipe for French toast. Always eat this with a protein since this alone does not have enough. We eat it with turkey sausage, chicken sausage, or eggs and reserve this as a weekend treat.

- 4 Slices Sprouted Grains Bread, Thawed
- ½ Cup Unsweetened Almond Milk
- 1 Large Egg
- 1 Tsp. Pure Vanilla Extract
- 1 Tbsp. Salted Butter
- ¼ Tsp. Ground Cinnamon

Makes 2 servings.

1. Heat a large pan to medium and add the butter, making sure it covers the entire bottom.
2. Using a glass pie dish (or equivalent), add the almond milk, egg, vanilla extract, and cinnamon and mix together with a fork.
3. Dip each piece of bread into the liquid mixture and then add to the heated pan.
4. Once all 4 pieces are added to the pan, add 3 wrist shakes of cinnamon to each piece of bread.
5. Flip after about 3-5 minutes or until nicely browned.
6. Cook an additional 3-5 minutes on the other side.
7. Serve with a separate protein.

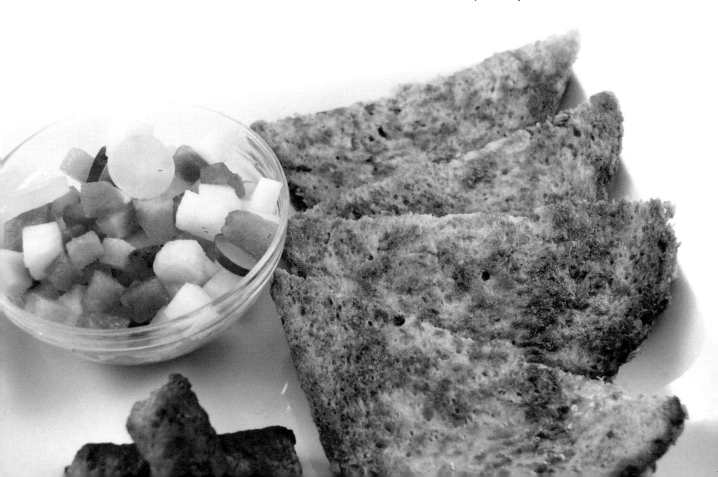

Protein-Packed Pancakes

You know we love protein so what better than protein-packed pancakes! We like our pancakes more salty than sweet, but the almond flour adds a bit of natural sweetness and the protein powder has sweetener in it as well.

Dry Ingredients:

- 2 Scoops Quality Vanilla Protein Powder (approx. 3 oz.)
- ¼ Cup Almond Flour, Blanched
- ¼ Cup Ground Golden Flaxseed
- ½ Tsp. Ground Cinnamon
- ½ Tsp. Aluminum-Free Baking Soda

Wet Ingredients:

- 2 Large Eggs*
- ½ Tbsp. Salted Butter
- ¼ Cup Unsweetened Almond Milk*
- ¼ Cup Coconut Oil
- ¼ Cup Low-Fat Cottage Cheese*
- ½ Tsp. Pure Vanilla Extract
- ¼ Tsp. Apple Cider Vinegar
- * Bring to room temperature

Makes 4 big pancakes or approximately 16 small pancakes.

1. In a large bowl, mix together the dry ingredients.
2. In a large bowl (preferably with a handle and a spout), mix together the wet ingredients with the exception of the eggs and the butter.
3. Pour the dry ingredients into the bowl of wet ingredients. Mix with a big spoon until smooth.
4. Beat the eggs in a small bowl with a fork and then fold the eggs into the mixture (do not over mix the eggs).
5. Using a large sized non-stick pan, add the butter and heat a burner to medium.
6. Once the butter is evenly melted, pour 4 large pancakes into the pan.
7. Once the pancakes start to form bubbles (about 3-4 minutes), flip over. Do not pat down the pancakes with the spatula.
8. Cook on the other side, about 3-4 minutes.
9. Remove and serve. If you prefer small pancakes (shown), use the rim of a cup to make cutouts.

tip

For all you waffle lovers, here is a high protein version that can be whipped up in no time! Just omit the cottage cheese and butter and then add in a ½ tbsp. of raw coconut nectar. Mix the wet and dry ingredients separately and then together (folding in the eggs) and pour into a waffle iron like you normally would. Makes 4 waffles.

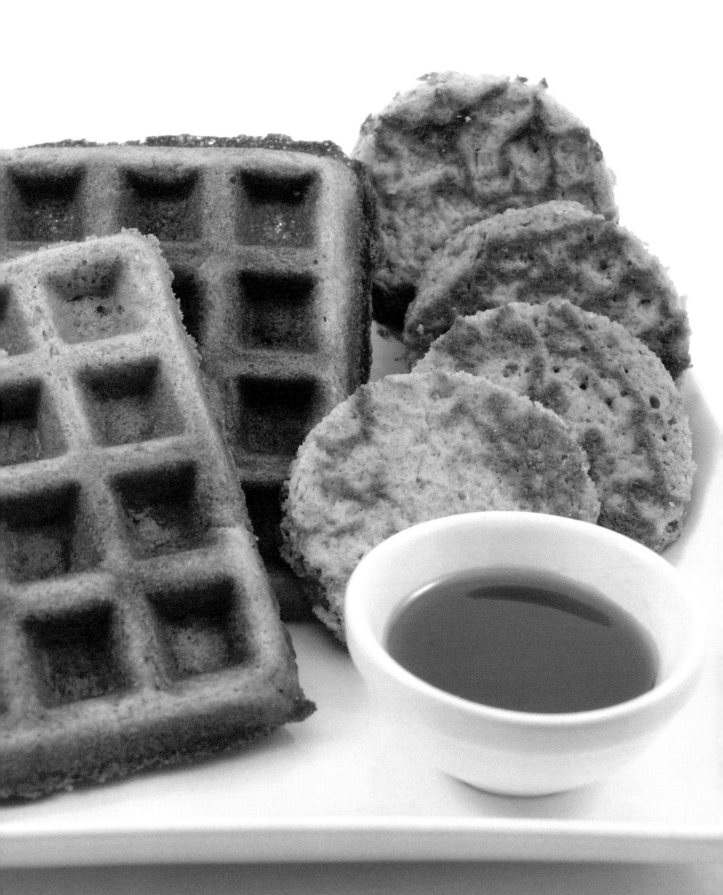

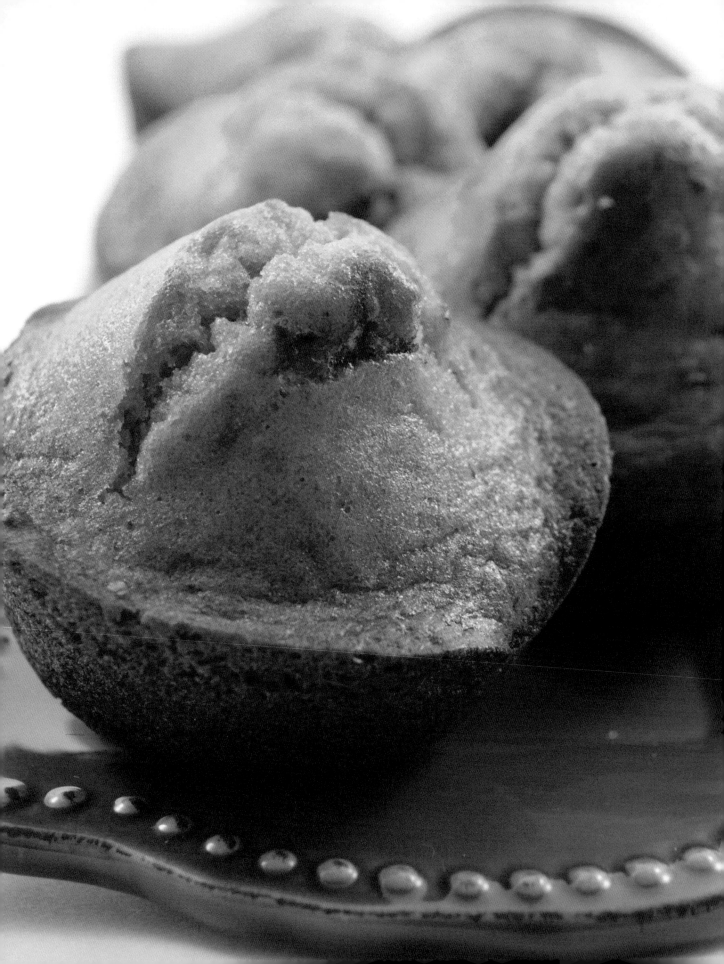

Higher-Protein Blueberry Muffins

Do you like blueberry muffins? Have you ever looked at the ingredients and the nutrition facts included in your favorite store bought muffins? You will likely be surprised at what you find. These are high in protein, moist, and can be a great addition to your breakfast or serve as a snack (and are great for traveling)!

Dry Ingredients:

- 1 Cup Almond Flour, Blanched
- 3 Scoops Quality Vanilla Protein Powder (approx. ⅔ cup)
- ⅓ Cup Ground Golden Flaxseed
- ½ Tsp. Pure Sea Salt
- ½ Tsp. Aluminum-Free Baking Soda

Wet Ingredients:

- 3 Large Eggs
- ¼ Cup Grapeseed Oil
- ⅓ Cup + 1 Tbsp. Raw Coconut Nectar
- 2 Tbsp. Unsweetened Applesauce
- 1 Cup Wild Blueberries, Frozen or Fresh

Makes 12 muffins.

1. Preheat the oven to 350 degrees.
2. In a large bowl, mix together the dry ingredients.
3. In a large bowl (preferably with a handle and a spout), mix together the wet ingredients with the exception of the blueberries.
4. Pour the dry ingredients into the bowl of wet ingredients. Mix with a big spoon until smooth.
5. Fold the blueberries into the mixture and set aside.
6. Take a muffin tray and spray with a non-stick spray or use your fingers to coat with coconut oil.
7. Pour the mixture into each of the muffin tins.
8. Place on the center rack and bake for 20 minutes or until golden brown.
9. Let stand for 5-10 minutes.
10. Serve.

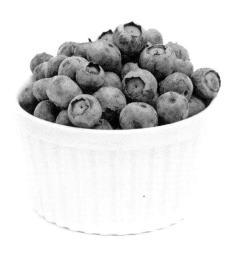

Higher-Protein Date (or Chocolate Chip) Muffins

My husband likes chocolate, but he equates chocolate chips with cookies so I had to come up with an alternative for him. Dates are a fruit and are very sweet and have a great texture when baked. This recipe gives you the option to interchange chocolate with dates. Enjoy!

Dry Ingredients:

- 1 Cup Almond Flour, Blanched
- 3 Scoops Quality Vanilla Protein Powder (approx. ⅔ cup)
- ⅓ Cup Ground Golden Flaxseed
- ½ Tsp. Pure Sea Salt
- ½ Tsp. Aluminum-Free Baking Soda

Wet Ingredients:

- 3 Large Eggs
- ¼ Cup Grapeseed Oil
- ⅓ Cup + 1 Tbsp. Raw Coconut Nectar
- ⅓ Pumpkin, Canned or Freshly Pureed
- ⅔ Cup Dates, Chopped and Pitted

Makes 12 muffins.

1. Preheat the oven to 350 degrees.
2. In a large bowl, mix together the dry ingredients.
3. In a large bowl (preferably with a handle and a spout), mix together the wet ingredients with the exception of the dates.
4. Pour the dry ingredients into the bowl of wet ingredients. Mix with a big spoon until smooth.
5. Fold the dates into the mixture and set aside.
6. Take a muffin tray and spray with a non-stick spray or use your fingers to coat with coconut oil.
7. Pour the mixture into each of the muffin tins.
8. Place on the center rack and bake for 20 minutes or until golden brown.
9. Let stand for 5-10 minutes.
10. Serve.

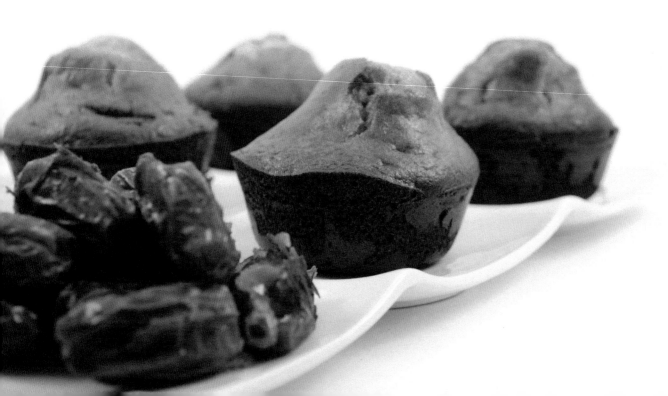

Carrot Zucchini Muffins

Yes, you read that right! Carrots actually have a natural sweetness to them and zucchini is a moisture agent and has a very neutral taste. So, trust me and try these out. You will not be disappointed and you will likely start looking at veggies differently!

Dry Ingredients:

- 1⅔ Cup Almond Flour, Blanched
- ⅓ Cup Ground Golden Flaxseed
- 1½ Tsp. Ground Cinnamon
- ½ Tsp. Pure Sea Salt
- ½ Tsp. Aluminum-Free Baking Soda

Wet Ingredients:

- 2 Large Eggs
- ⅔ Cup Finely Chopped Carrots, Outer Layer Removed
- ½ Cup Finely Chopped Zucchini, Outer Layer Removed
- ⅓ Cup Raw Coconut Nectar
- ¼ Cup Grapeseed Oil

Makes 12 muffins.

1. Preheat the oven to 350 degrees.
2. Using a large bowl, mix together the dry ingredients.
3. Using a large bowl (preferably with a handle and a spout), mix together the wet ingredients with the exception of the carrots and zucchini.
4. Pour the dry ingredients into the bowl of wet ingredients. Mix with a big spoon until smooth.
5. Fold the carrots and zucchini into the mixture and set aside.
6. Take a muffin tray and spray with a non-stick spray or use your fingers to coat with coconut oil.
7. Pour the mixture into each of the muffin tins.
8. Place on the center rack and bake for 25-30 minutes or until golden brown.
9. Let stand for 20 minutes.
10. Serve.

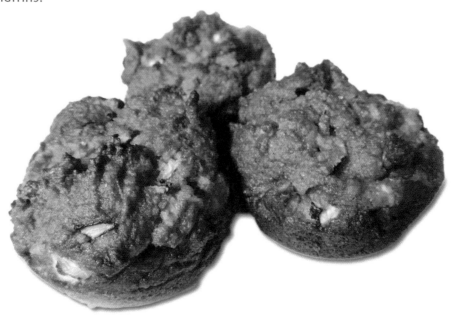

Chocolate Blueberry Kale Shake

Talk about a healthy shake! With kale and blueberries, this is packed full of antioxidants! The chocolate protein powder makes this high in protein and the ground flaxseed gives you the healthy fats. This is a great way to disguise kale while reaping all its benefits!

- 1 Cup Fresh Kale, Packed
- 1 Cup Unsweetened Almond Milk
- ½ Cup Wild Blueberries, Frozen
- ½ Cup Ice
- 1 Scoop High Quality Chocolate Protein Powder (approx. 1.5 oz.)
- 1 Tbsp. Ground Golden Flaxseed

Makes 1-2 servings.

1. Using a blender*, add each of the ingredients.
2. Place the lid on the blender and blend away until the shake is fully mixed and has a shake consistency.
3. Serve immediately.

*If you found kale in your shake, you need to invest in a blender that can liquefy vegetables. I use a NutriBullet® system.

Avocado Chocolate Protein Shake

I know you may be skeptical, but I think you will be pleasantly surprised when you realize how easy this is to drink. Avocados are very nutritious and have a great consistency. The first time I gave this to my husband, he reluctantly took it from me and gave me that, "do you really want me to try this" look. After the first sip, his facial expression started to change and before I knew it, he drank the entire cup!

- 1 Hass Avocado, Pitted
- 1 Cup Unsweetened Almond Milk
- ½ Cup Ice
- 1 Scoop High Quality Chocolate Protein Powder (approx. 1.5 oz.)

Makes 1 serving.

1. Using a spoon, scoop out the bright green avocado meat and place in a blender and then add the remaining ingredients.
2. Discard the outer avocado shell.
3. Place the lid on the blender and blend away until the shake is fully mixed and has a shake consistency.
4. Serve immediately.

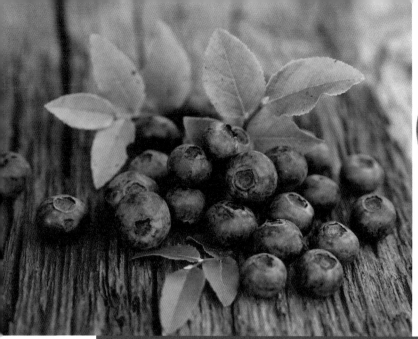

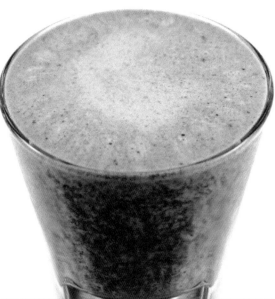

tip

Looking for a simple chocolate/banana shake recipe? Just omit the kale and blueberries and add a banana. For a thicker consistency, use a frozen banana. For those of you new to freezing bananas, remove the peel before placing in the freezer. Just wrap it with foil and parchment paper-in-one (with the parchment side touching the banana) and you will save yourself a lot of headache when trying to remove a frozen peel!

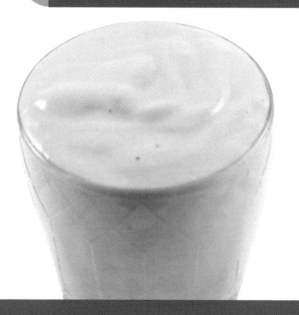

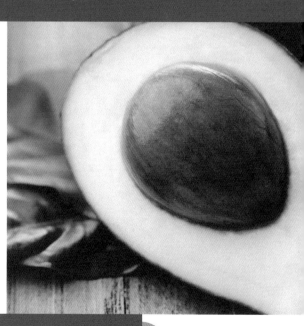

Do you love Reese® cups? I have a shake for that! For a simple chocolate/ peanut butter shake, omit the avocado and add in 2 tbsp. organic unsweetened peanut butter, almond butter, or sunbutter. You will love me for this!

tip

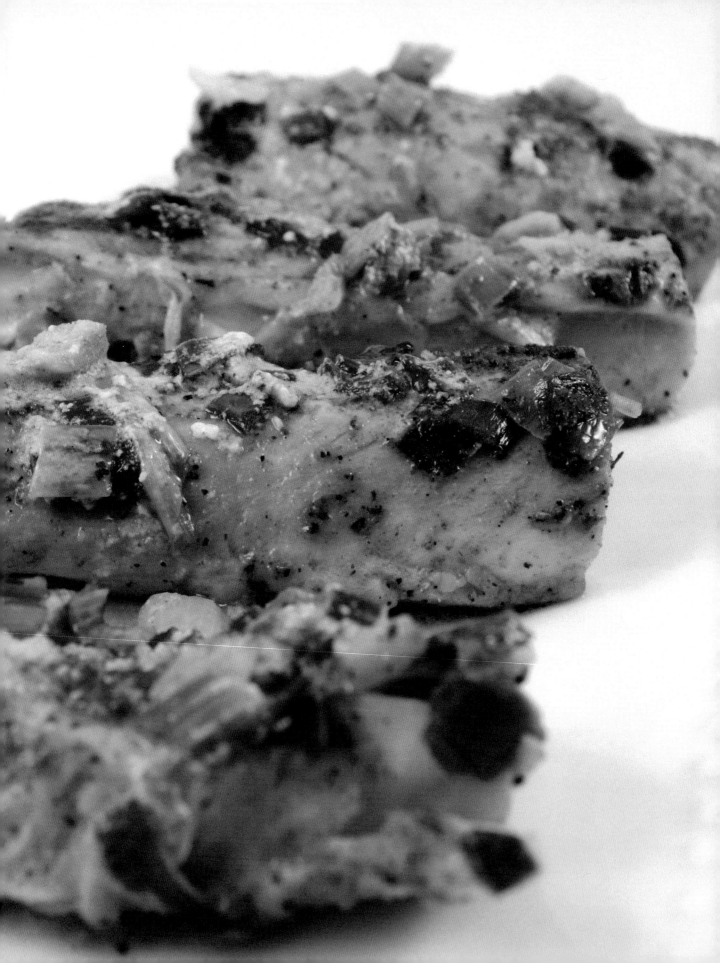

lunch/dinner entrées and sides

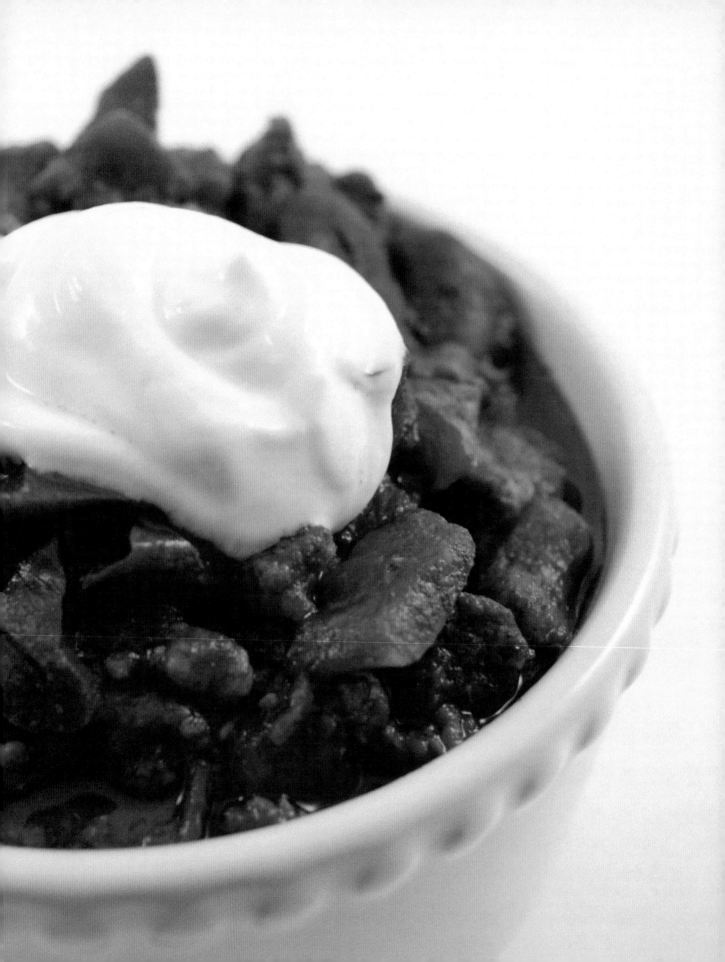

Buffalo Bean Veggie Slow Cooker Chili

This chili recipe takes about 10 minutes to prepare and is very hearty. Buffalo (also called Bison) is higher in protein than other meats. I think it tastes better than beef so if you are reluctant, don't be! You can always substitute ground beef, ground turkey, or even shredded chicken.

- 1 LB Ground Buffalo
- 2 Cups Peppers and Onions, Cut in Strips
- 15 oz. Can Diced Tomatoes
- 15 oz. Can Tomato Sauce
- 15 oz. Can Black Beans, Drained and Rinsed
- 15 oz. Can Kidney Beans, Drained and Rinsed
- 1.25 oz. Packet Quality Taco Seasoning*
- 1 Tbsp. Pure Unsweetened Cocoa
- ½ Tbsp. Chili Powder

Makes 6 servings.

1. Heat a large skillet to med-high and sauté the ground buffalo and once the meat is browned, drain any grease.
2. Add all ingredients to a slow cooker.
3. Using a large spoon, stir all ingredients together.
4. Cover and set to high and cook for 3 hours.
5. Serve over lettuce or rice with a dollop of Greek yogurt and slices of avocado.

*Review the package and make sure you recognize all the ingredients. I use Wick Fowler's®, which includes ground chili peppers, salt, onion, cumin, garlic, and oregano.

tip

To save time, use a frozen pepper/onion mix. Just run it under cold water and massage it to break iced up clumps and then throw it in the slow cooker.

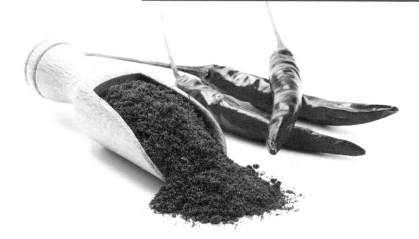

Grain-Free Turkey Meatloaf

This recipe was created when my husband and I completed a twenty-day detox-eating plan (elimination of sugars, grains, dairy, and other inflammatory foods), but I have kept it as part of our normal menu. Serve with *cauliflower mashed "potatoes"* (page 74) or *sweet potato smashed* (page 76) and your favorite greens.

- 1 LB Ground Turkey
- 8 oz. Can Tomato Sauce, Halved
- ¼ Cup Ground Golden Flaxseed
- 1 Large Egg
- ½ Tbsp. Onion Powder
- 1 Tsp. Organic Worcestershire Sauce
- ½ Tsp. Garlic Powder
- ½ Tsp. Pure Sea Salt

Makes 4 servings.

1. Preheat the oven to 400 degrees and cover a large baking sheet with foil and parchment paper-in-one (with the foil facing down so it does not touch the food). Set aside.

2. Set aside half of the can of tomato sauce (4 oz.).

3. Combine the remaining ingredients together in a large bowl and massage with your hands until evenly distributed.

4. Place the meat mixture on the baking sheet and form a rounded rectangle.

5. Pour the remaining tomato sauce on top of the meatloaf so it is evenly dispersed.

6. Bake uncovered for 35-40 minutes.

7. Serve.

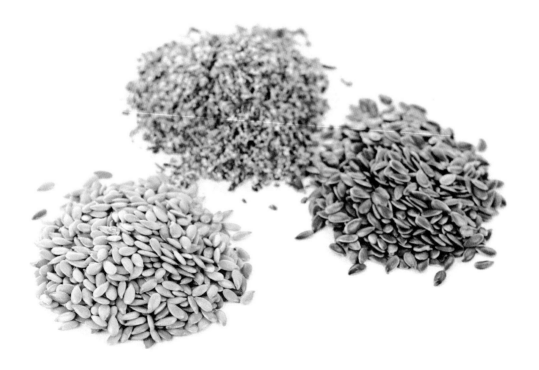

Something Like Goulash

This meal hits the spot when you are looking for a pasta meal equivalent. By pre making the rice and chicken, this can be whipped up in no time!

- 2½ Cups Brown Rice, Cooked (approx. 1 cup uncooked)
- 1 LB Chicken Breast, Cooked and Cubed
- ½ LB Mild Italian Chicken Sausage, Casing Removed
- 1 Med. Zucchini, Chopped Finely with Ends Removed
- 2 Med. Yellow Squash, Chopped Finely with Ends Removed
- 8 Oz. Baby Bella Mushrooms, Chopped Finely
- 24 oz. Jar Organic Olive Oil, Basil, and Garlic Pasta Sauce
- 1 Tbsp. Extra Virgin Olive Oil (EVOO)
- ¼ Tsp. Pure Sea Salt
- ⅛ Tsp. Ground Black Pepper

Makes approximately 6 servings.

1. Heat a large skillet to medium and then add the EVOO, covering the bottom completely.
2. Add the zucchini, yellow squash, and mushrooms.
3. Sauté until soft, approximately 6 minutes stirring half way through.
4. Heat a medium skillet to med-high and add the chicken sausage and cook like you would ground turkey or beef.
5. Heat a large pot to med-high and add all the ingredients together, stirring frequently until heated (approx. 8 minutes).
6. Serve.

tip

Roast a large batch of the zucchini and squash in advance (you will need approx. 1 cup of each for this recipe) and reduce the cooking time even more. Have leftover vegetables from the night before? Throw them in, too!

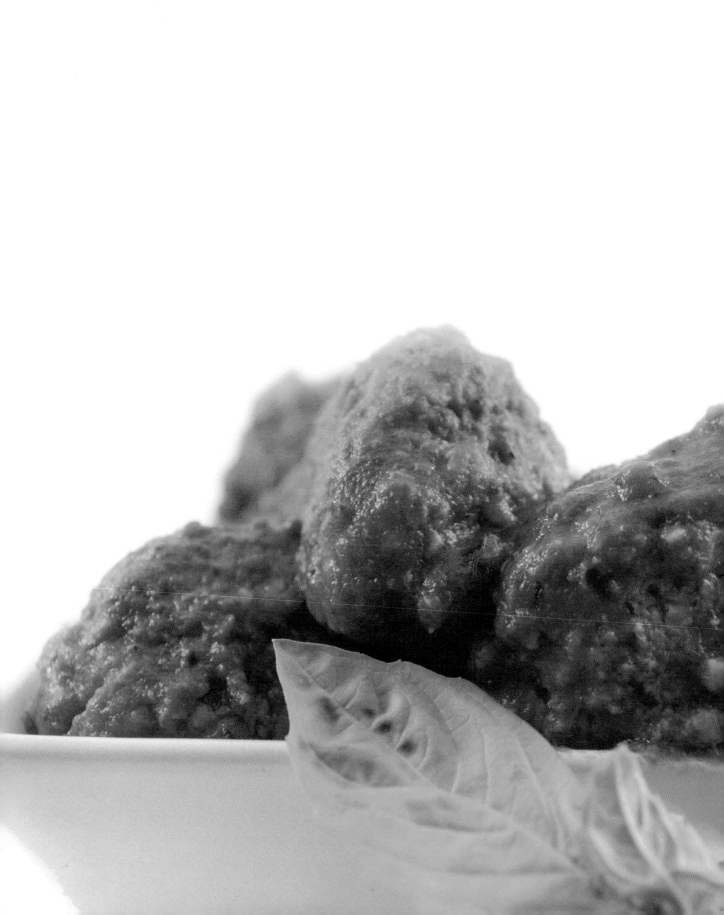

Turkey Zucchini Meatballs

Zucchini is extremely versatile and can be added to almost anything due to its neutral flavor and its moisture properties.

- 1 LB Ground Turkey
- 2 Large Eggs
- ½ Cup *Better Breadcrumbs* (page 86)
- ⅓ Cup Zucchini, Minced with Skin Removed
- 2 Tbsp. Ground Golden Flaxseed
- 2 Tbsp. Parmesan Cheese
- 2 Tbsp. Unsweetened Almond Milk
- ½ Tbsp. Italian Seasoning

Makes approximately 14 meatballs.

1. Combine all ingredients in a large bowl and massage with your hands.
2. Form into balls and add to a large pot.
3. Add your favorite organic red sauce and make sure all meatballs are covered with sauce.
4. Heat the stovetop to low, cover the pot, and simmer for 1 hour. Stir halfway through.
5. Serve.

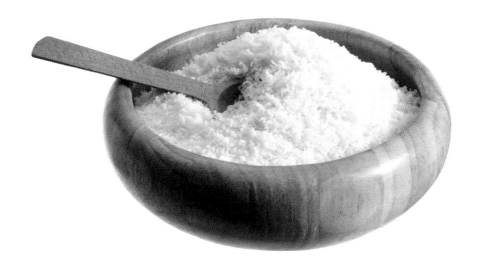

Hybrid Stuffed Peppers

This is a hybrid recipe because it is a combination of my mom's recipe and my mother-in-law's recipe with a few of my own elements.

- 4 Med-Large Peppers
- 1 LB Ground Turkey
- 1 Med. Onion, Minced
- 2 Stalks Celery, Minced
- 2½ Cups Brown Rice, Cooked
  (approx. 1 cup uncooked)
- 15 Oz. Can Tomato Sauce
- 1 Tsp. Garlic Powder
- 2 Tsp. Organic Worcestershire Sauce
- 1½ Tsp. Pure Sea Salt
- ½ Tsp. Ground Black Pepper

Makes 4 servings.

1. Preheat the oven to 350 degrees.
2. Cut off the top of the peppers and deseed them.
3. Bring a large pot of water to a boil and drop the peppers in for 5 minutes (make sure they are submerged). Remove from the pot (be careful, they will be hot) and shake out the water. Place the peppers in a glass-baking dish.
4. Heat a large skillet to med-high and sauté the ground turkey and the onion and once the meat is browned, drain any grease.
5. In a large bowl, mix together the turkey, onion, and cooked rice and add the chopped celery, garlic powder, salt, and pepper.
6. Pour the tomato sauce into the bowl, reserving just enough to make 4 big spoonfuls over the finished peppers.
7. Add the Worcestershire sauce and mix everything together.
8. Spoon mixture into each of the peppers.
9. Add a spoonful of the remaining sauce onto each of the peppers.
10. Place in the oven on the center rack and bake for 35 minutes, uncovered.
11. Serve.

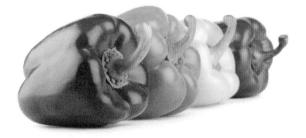

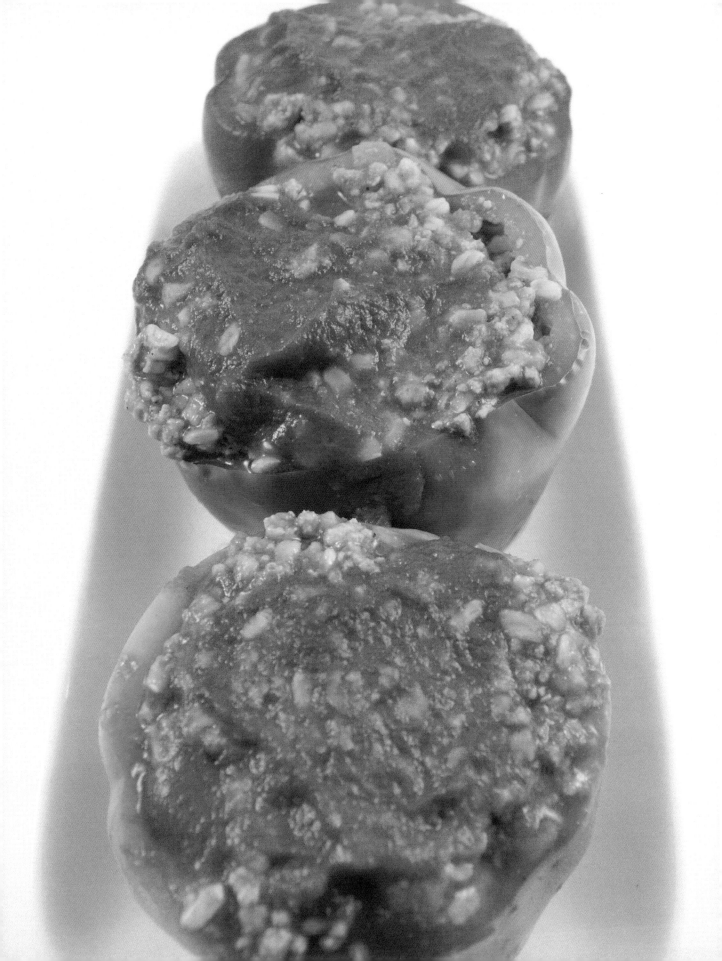

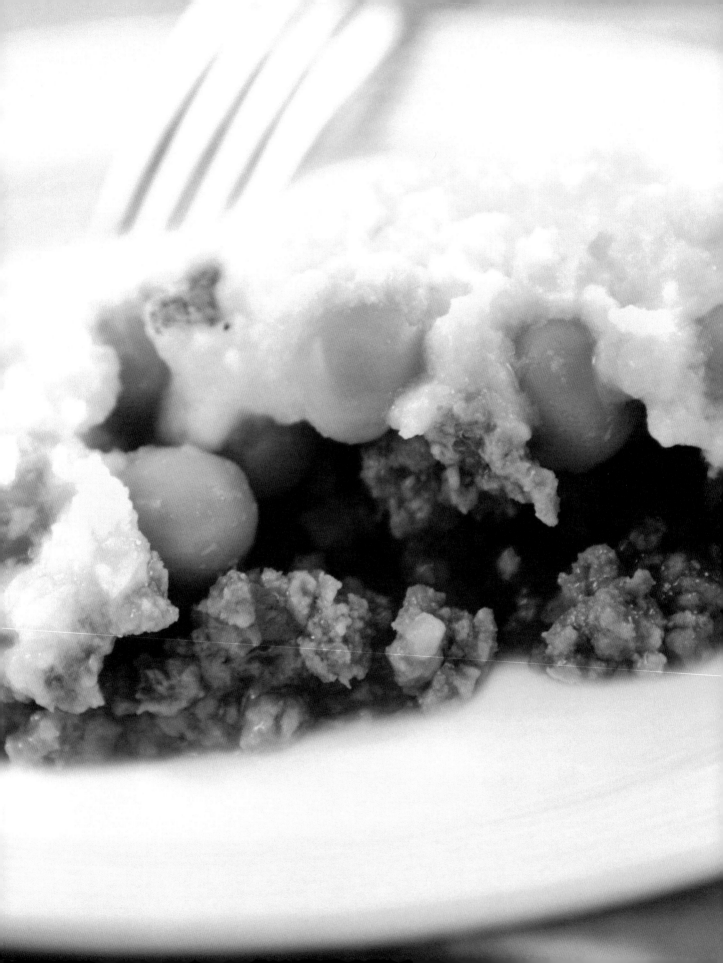

Shepherd's Cauliflower "Pie"

If you are looking for comfort food then this is it! However, you do not have to feel guilty about eating this dish. It has half potatoes and half cauliflower and uses homemade brown gravy.

- 1⅓ LB Organic Beef
- ½ Large Onion, Minced
- 1 Cup Baby Bella Mushrooms, Minced
- 15 oz. Can Corn or Green Peas, Drained and Rinsed
- Batch *Smashed "Taters"* (page 75)
- Batch *Cauliflower Mashed "Potatoes"* (page 74)

Brown Gravy Ingredients (page 95)*:*

- 1 Cup Organic Beef Broth
- 1 Tbsp. Salted Butter
- 1 Tbsp. Organic Cornstarch
- 1 Tsp. Pure Sea Salt
- ½ Tsp. Garlic Powder
- ¼ Tsp. Onion Powder
- ⅛ Tsp. Ground Black Pepper

Makes 4-5 servings.

1. Preheat the oven to 375 degrees.
2. Heat a large skillet to med-high and sauté the ground beef and the onion. Once the meat is browned, drain the grease. Add the beef to a large glass-baking dish and make sure it completely covers the bottom. Add the mushrooms on top of the beef.
3. To make the brown gravy, use a fork to mix together the broth and the cornstarch in a small bowl. Once all clumps are gone, pour in the remaining ingredients and mix.
4. Return the skillet to the stovetop, add the butter, and melt.
5. Pour all the liquid in the pan and stir continuously until it thickens.
6. Evenly pour the gravy on top of the mushrooms and then add the corn on top of the mushrooms.
7. Combine the *smashed "taters"* and the *cauliflower mashed "potatoes."*
8. Add the cauliflower potato mixture to the baking dish and spread so you no longer see the corn, mushrooms, or beef.
9. Take a large fork and pierce about 8 spots in the dish to allow the juices to move through.
10. Place in the oven on the center rack and bake for 25 minutes, uncovered.
11. Serve.

Not Quite Chicken Pot "Pie"

After several attempts at making traditional "pot pie," this recipe resembles a combination of my mom's chicken divan and traditional "pot pie." No matter what it is called, it is delicious! This recipe takes a bit of time to make so I recommend pre cooking the chicken and just pull it out when you need it. As you can see, I do not use cream of chicken or mushroom soup because of all the preservatives and unfamiliar ingredients.

Main Ingredients:

- 3 Large Chicken Breasts, Cooked and Cubed
- 1 Cup Zucchini, Cubed
- 1 Cup Broccoli, Stems Removed
- 1 Cup Red Onion, Chopped
- 1 Cup Baby Bella Mushrooms, Chopped
- 1 Tbsp. Salted Butter
- Salt and Pepper

Liquid Ingredients:

- 1½ Cup Organic Chicken Broth, Low Sodium
- ¾ Cup Unsweetened Almond Milk
- 1 Tbsp. Organic Cornstarch
- 1 Tsp. Pure Sea Salt
- ¾ Tsp. Garlic Powder
- ¾ Tsp. Onion Powder
- ½ Tsp. Ground Parsley
- ¼ Tsp. Ground Dill
- ⅛ Tsp. Ground Black Pepper

Topping Ingredients:

- 1 Cup Almond Flour, Blanched
- ½ Cup Ground Golden Flaxseed
- ¼ Cup Grapeseed Oil
- 2 Tbsp. Unsweetened Almond Milk
- 1 Tbsp. Ground Parsley
- ½ Tsp. Pure Sea Salt
- ½ Tsp. Aluminum-Free Baking Soda

Makes 4-5 servings.

1. Preheat the oven to 350 degrees.
2. Heat a large skillet to med-high and then add the butter and melt, making sure it evenly coats the bottom of the pan.
3. Add the red onions and mushrooms and sauté for about 6-8 minutes and then transfer to a large glass-baking dish. Add the remaining main ingredients to the baking dish. Stir the mixture so that it is evenly distributed in the dish.
4. Return the skillet to the stovetop.
5. Combine the broth and the cornstarch in a small bowl and mix until all clumps are gone and then pour into the skillet.
6. Add the remaining liquid ingredients to the skillet.
7. Stir continuously until the liquid starts to become a bit thicker. Remove and pour into the baking dish.
8. In a large bowl, combine all the topping ingredients and stir with a large spoon.
9. Grab a handful of the mixture with your hands and drop pieces on top of the baking dish.
10. Repeat until the baking dish is covered in "crumbles."
11. Place in the oven on the center rack and bake for 20 minutes or until the topping is golden and crunchy.
12. Serve.

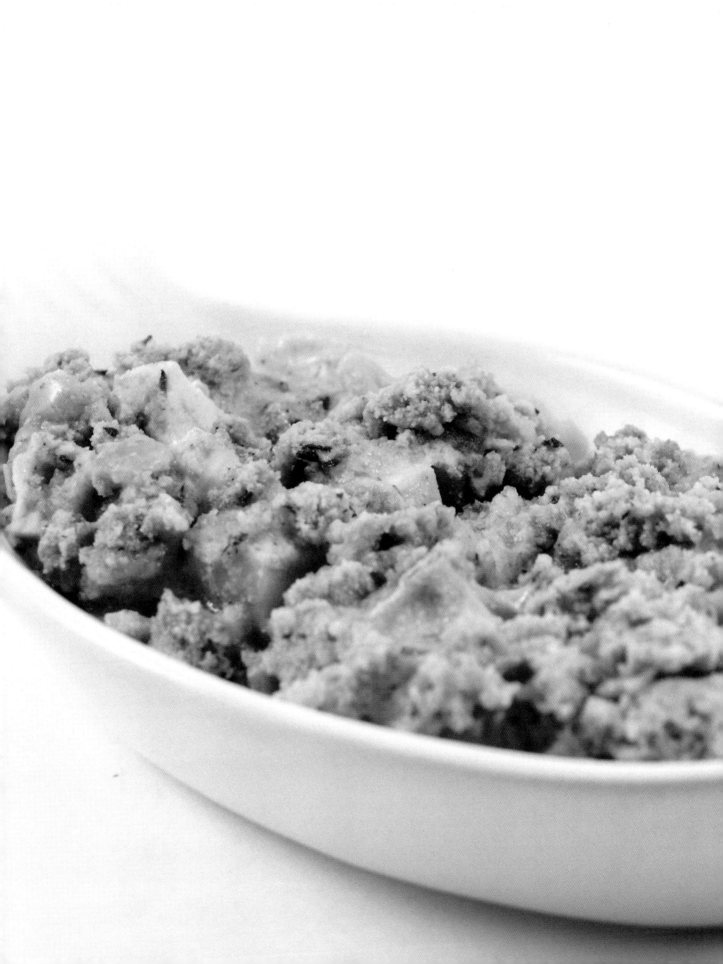

Mom's Chicken Veggie "Fried" Rice

This can be customized to your liking by using different vegetables or using shrimp instead of chicken. When you think of traditional "fried" rice, rice is the main ingredient and the veggies and meat are secondary. In this recipe, the chicken and veggies are the main ingredients and the rice is secondary. What does this mean? You get the benefits from the vegetables and chicken and you satisfy your craving without spiking your blood sugar.

- 2½ Cups Brown Rice, Cooked
  (approx. 1 cup uncooked)
- 2 Large Eggs
- 3 Cups Chicken, Cooked and Chopped
  (approx. 1.5 lb.)
- 1 Cup Carrots, Finely Chopped
- 1 Cup Bean Sprouts
- 1 Cup Mushrooms, Chopped
- ½ Cup Celery, Finely Chopped
- 1 Med. Onion, Finely Chopped
- 2 Tbsp. Organic Low Sodium Soy Sauce
- 2 Tbsp. Salted Butter
- ½ Tsp. Pure Sea Salt
- ¼ Tsp. Ground Black Pepper

Makes approximately 6 servings.

1. Heat a large skillet to med-high and then add the butter.
2. Once the butter is melted and covers the skillet completely, add the carrots, celery, and onion.
3. Sauté until soft, approximately 6 minutes stirring half way through.
4. While the vegetables are cooking, bring another burner to med-high heat and spray a small pan with a non-stick spray. Add the eggs and fry them up.
5. Add the mushrooms and bean sprouts to the large skillet, stir, and cook for an additional 5 minutes.
6. Add the chicken, rice, and eggs to the large skillet and stir.
7. Add the soy sauce, salt, and pepper to the large skillet and stir until everything is mixed well and heated.
8. Serve.

tip

To save time, pre cook the chicken breasts and rice and refrigerate until you need it. If you are not going to use the cooked chicken within 2-3 days then use a vacuum seal system and freeze it. To save even more time, rely on your food processor to finely chop the carrots, celery, and onion.

Eat this dish with chopsticks. Not only is it a test of coordination, it will take you longer to eat so you likely will eat less, but feel completely satisfied.

Jeff's Cilantro-Lime-Inspired Salmon

A work colleague of mine gave me this recipe and I made minor tweaks. If you like cilantro, you will enjoy the salmon when it is made, but also the experience of making it because of cilantro's great aroma. Salmon is full of the healthy fats and we eat it about twice per week.

- 3 Large Wild-Caught Salmon Fillets
- 2 Cups Fresh Cilantro, Chopped
- 2 Med. Limes
- 1½ Tbsp. Salted Butter
- Salt, Pepper, and Garlic Powder
- Raw Coconut Sugar (Granulated Powder)

Makes 3-4 servings.

1. Add the salmon fillets to a plastic storage bag, squeeze the limes, and add the cilantro.
2. Close the bag and massage to make sure each fillet is evenly coated with the lime and the cilantro.
3. Place in the refrigerator for 30 minutes.
4. Pull the bag of fish from the refrigerator and place on a plate. Sprinkle each fillet with salt, pepper, and garlic powder.
5. Heat a large skillet to med-high and then add the butter, melting it until it covers the bottom completely.
6. Add the fillets (cilantro bits and all) to the pan with the skin side up. Flip after approx. 5 minutes.
7. Cook for another 5 minutes. Depending on the size of the fillets, you may need to cook longer until no longer pink in the middle.
8. Remove the skin, which comes off easily.
9. Sprinkle with the coconut sugar.
10. Serve.

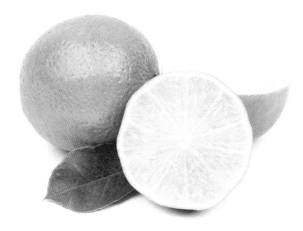

Dad's White Sauce Fish

My dad took such pride in making this recipe and it was the joy he had that I now have when I cook. I stayed away from making this recipe for a long time because it used half and half or evaporated milk to make the "white sauce." After a little bit of experimenting, I was able to come up with a healthier alternative, but the white sauce is not so white but neither was my dad's now that I think about it!

- 4 Med-Large Wild-Caught Mahi Fillets
- ¼ Cup White Wine
- ¼ Cup + 2 Tbsp. 1% Milk
- 3 oz. Container Green Onions, Chopped
- 2 Tbsp. Plain Greek Yogurt
- 2 Tbsp. Salted Butter
- 1 Med. Lemon, Cut in Half
- Chef Paul Prudhomme® Blackened Redfish Magic Seasoning

Makes 4 servings.

1. Heat a large skillet to med-high and then add the butter, melting it until it covers the bottom completely.
2. Add the onions and sauté for about 3 minutes.
3. Apply a generous portion of the seasoning to both sides of the fish and add to the skillet. Cook for about 4-5 minutes on each side.
4. Fish is done once it is white and flaky. Remove once done, but leave onion shards.
5. Add the wine and squeeze each lemon half into the skillet. Stir.
6. In a measuring cup, mix together the milk and yogurt and then add to the skillet. Bring to a boil.
7. Stir continuously, about 3-4 minutes.
8. Pour the sauce over the fish.
9. Serve.

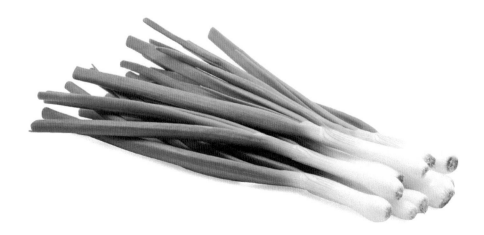

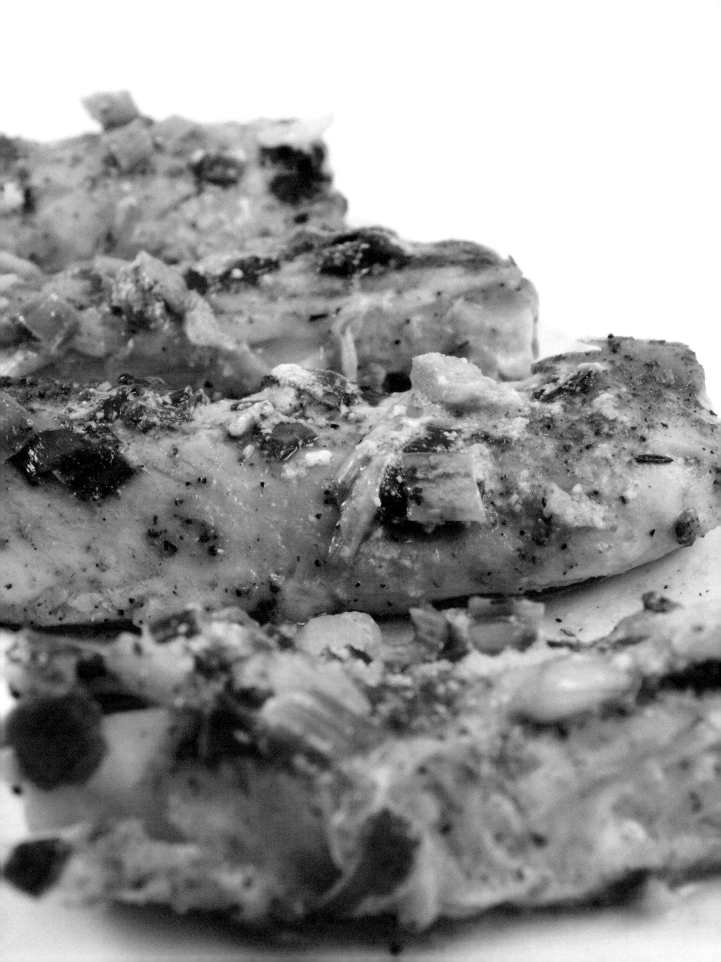

No-Noodle Lasagna

I rely on zucchini and eggplant to serve as the "noodles" in this dish so you will get full quicker and stay full longer than with traditional white pasta recipes. This takes a bit of time to make so I recommend pre making the ground turkey.

- 1 LB Ground Turkey, Cooked with ½ Cup Minced Onions
- 3 Med. Zucchini, Skin Removed
- 1 Eggplant (approx. 1.25 lb.)
- 24 oz. Jar Organic Olive Oil, Basil, and Garlic Pasta Sauce
- ½ Cup Quality Mozzarella Cheese, Shredded
- ¼ Cup Quality Parmesan Cheese, Grated
- Italian Seasonings

Makes 4-5 servings.

Directions:

1. Preheat the oven to 400 degrees and cover 2 baking sheets with foil and parchment paper-in-one (with the foil facing down so it does not touch the food).
2. Cut the zucchini in half and then make ¼ inch slices so you end up with thin noodle "strips."
3. Cut the top and bottom of the eggplant and discard. Cut the eggplant lengthwise in ¼ inch-thick cuts so you end up with approx. 6-8 rectangular pieces.
4. To help reduce the bitterness that eggplant can have, place eggplant (you may need 2 baking sheets) on a baking sheet and salt both sides. Set aside for 30 minutes.
5. Once the 30 minutes is up, run each eggplant under water, removing the salt from each and then dry with a paper towel.
6. Arrange the eggplant on the lined baking sheet so they are not touching. Sprinkle with Italian seasoning.
7. Arrange the zucchini on the other lined baking sheet so they are not touching. Sprinkle with Italian seasoning.
8. Place the baking sheet with eggplant on the center rack and roast for 15-20 minutes.
9. Place the baking sheet with zucchini on the lower rack and roast for 15 minutes.
10. Reduce the oven to 375 degrees.
11. Pour about ½ cup of the pasta sauce into the bottom of a large glass-baking dish. Use a small spoon to spread it around to cover the bottom completely.
12. Layer the zucchini, then the eggplant, another layer of sauce, the ground turkey, another layer of sauce, the Parmesan cheese, more zucchini, and then the remaining sauce.
13. Place in the oven on the center rack and bake for 20 minutes.
14. Remove and sprinkle the mozzarella cheese so it evenly covers the baking dish.
15. Place back in the oven and bake for 10 minutes or until the cheese is melted with a touch of brown.
16. Serve.

Eggplant Tomato "Parm" Alternative

I love Eggplant Parmesan so I've created an alternative that is healthier, quicker to make and best of all, requires minimal cleanup! This can be your primary dish, a side, or an appetizer! I usually serve this with baked chicken and a spoonful of sauce.

- 1 Eggplant (approx. 1.25 lbs.)
- 2 Large Premium Tomatoes
- ½ Cup Organic Olive Oil, Basil, and Garlic Pasta Sauce
- ⅓ Cup Quality Mozzarella Cheese, Shredded

Makes 4 servings as a side item.

Directions:

1. Preheat the oven to 400 degrees.
2. Cut the top and bottom of the eggplant and discard.
3. Make ¼ inch-thick cuts lengthwise so you have long eggplant "sheets."
4. Discard the 2 end pieces that have skin on them.
5. Cut each eggplant sheet in half so you end up with approx. 12 squares.
6. To help reduce the bitterness that eggplant can have, place the 12 squares (you may need 2 baking sheets) on a large baking sheet and salt both sides. Set aside for 30 minutes.
7. Once the 30 minutes is up, run each square under water, removing the salt from each, and then dry with a paper towel.
8. Cover a large baking sheet with foil and parchment paper-in-one (with the foil facing down so it does not touch the food).
9. Arrange the squares on the baking sheet so they are not touching.
10. Using a small spoon, spoon sauce onto each square.
11. Cut the tomatoes about ¼ inch thick so you end up with approx. 12 slices.
12. Place each tomato slice on each eggplant square. Shake a small amount of salt on each tomato.
13. Place in the oven on the center rack and bake for 20 minutes.
14. Remove from the oven and add another small spoonful of sauce on each of the tomatoes. Add a double pinch of cheese on each tomato.
15. Place back in the oven for 10 minutes or until the cheese is melted with a touch of brown.
16. Serve.

Cauliflower Mashed "Potatoes"

I know I have "potatoes" in the title, but guess what? You will not find any potatoes in this recipe! Cauliflower is very versatile and can actually be served up as an alternative to mashed potatoes. It takes no time at all to make and eliminates the need for a separate "starch," which means less time in the kitchen! If you are on the fence then I suggest doing a hybrid batch first (half potatoes and half cauliflower).

• 1 Cauliflower Head, Cut into Chunks with Greens Removed
• ½ Cup Plain Greek Yogurt
• ½ Tsp. Pure Sea Salt
• ½ Tsp. Garlic Powder
• ¼ Tsp. Ground Black Pepper

Makes 3-4 servings.

1. Start by taking the yogurt out of the refrigerator to allow it to get close to room temperature.
2. Pour all the cauliflower pieces into a steamer.
3. Fill a pot up with water (about 2-3 inches, leaving enough room for the steamer to sit on top of the water without touching).
4. Preheat the stovetop to high heat and then add the pot.
5. Add a couple of shakes of pure sea salt and bring the water to a boil.
6. Once it starts boiling, take your steamer and place on top of the boiling pot. Cover the steamer.
7. Continue boiling for 10 minutes, steaming the cauliflower.
8. Pour the steamed cauliflower into a food processor.
9. Add the yogurt and the spices. Blend until it has the consistency of mashed potatoes.
10. Serve.

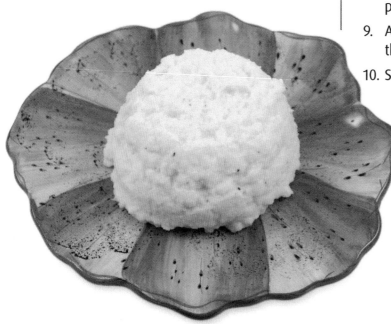

Smashed "Taters"

My dad taught me how to make mashed potatoes and he would call them "taters." Peeling potatoes takes a long time so I leave the skins on hence the "smashed" term. The skins are full of nutrients and you barely notice them in the final product. With just a few changes, these smashed potatoes are healthier than traditional mashed potatoes and are still very tasty.

- 2 Med. Potatoes, Yukon Gold or Idaho
- ½ Cup Organic Low Sodium Chicken Broth or 1% Milk
- ¼ Cup Plain Greek Yogurt
- 1 Tbsp. Salted Butter
- ¼ Tsp. Pure Sea Salt
- ⅛ Tsp. Ground Black Pepper

Makes 3-4 servings.

1. Take the Greek yogurt out of the refrigerator (or milk, if using) to get close to room temperature.
2. Wash the potatoes, cut into medium chunks, and then add to a medium sized pot.
3. Fill the pot with water so that the water is about ½ inch above the potatoes. Add 4 shakes of salt to the pot (in addition to the ¼ tsp. salt above).
4. Preheat the stovetop to high heat and add the pot.
5. Bring the pot to a boil and then set a timer for 15 minutes.
6. Pour the cooked potatoes into a strainer, but do not run the potatoes under water. You want them to be as hot as possible to melt the butter.
7. Add the butter to the empty pot. Pour the drained potatoes back into the pot.
8. Add the yogurt and broth or milk. Use a hand mixer and mix on high until all chunks are gone.
9. Add the salt and pepper and continue to mix until it is a whipped consistency.
10. Serve.

Sweet Potato Smashed

Sweet potatoes are full of minerals and nutrients and are an excellent complex carbohydrate. My fitness fanatic loves his sweet potatoes "sweet" so I build on the potato's natural attributes. Like the *mashed "taters"* (page 75), these are made with the skins to save time and to maximize the nutritional benefits.

• 3 Med. Sweet Potatoes

• ½ Cup Unsweetened Almond Milk

• ½ Tsp. Ground Cinnamon

• 2 Tsp. Coconut Nectar

Makes 5-6 servings.

1. Wash the potatoes, cut into medium chunks and then add to a medium sized pot.

2. Fill the pot with water so that the water is about ½ inch above the potatoes. Add 4 shakes of salt to the pot.

3. Preheat the stovetop to high heat and add the pot.

4. Bring the pot to a boil and then set a timer for 15 minutes.

5. Pour the cooked potatoes into a strainer, but do not run the potatoes under water.

6. Pour the drained potatoes back into the pot.

7. Add the almond milk. Use a hand mixer and mix on high until all chunks are gone.

8. Add the cinnamon and nectar and continue to mix until it is a whipped consistency. Sprinkle with additional cinnamon for a nice color.

9. Serve.

tip

Do you have leftover baked potatoes from a previous meal? Then use them in lieu of boiling new ones! Just cut up the baked potatoes (skins and all) and heat them up and then add the remaining ingredients and mix away!

Zucchini Fritters

My kindergarten teacher gave me this recipe (yes, I still stay in touch with her). I have made minor adjustments to make it a little healthier. Feel free to use different veggies.

- 1 Cup Zucchini, Skinned and Finely Chopped (or Grated)
- ¼ Cup Almond Flour, Blanched
- 2 Tbsp. Extra Virgin Olive Oil (EVOO)
- 2 Tbsp. Parmesan Cheese
- 1 Large Egg
- ¼ Tsp. Pure Sea Salt
- ¼ Tsp. Ground Black Pepper

Makes approximately 5 small fritters.

1. Mix together all the ingredients with the exception of the EVOO.
2. Heat a large non-stick pan over medium heat.
3. Add the EVOO and make sure you coat the entire pan.
4. Spoon the mixture onto the heated pan and make approximately 5 fritters.
5. Cook on both sides for approximately 4 minutes each or until golden brown. Repeat with any leftover batter.
6. Serve.

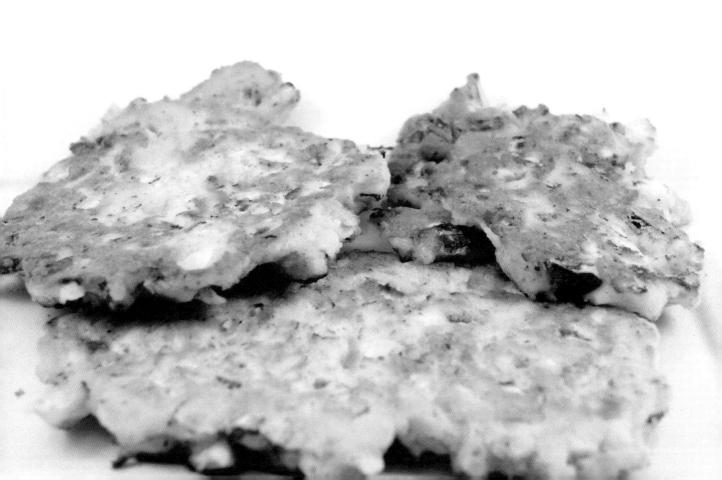

Cauliflower "Rice"

Cauliflower served as rice? Yes, you read that right! This vegetable has the ability to change its texture to resemble many family favorites. Like the *cauliflower mashed "potatoes"* (page 74), if you are hesitant then just start by making half rice and half cauliflower.

- 1 Cauliflower Head, Cut into Chunks with Greens Removed
- ½ Cup Celery, Chopped (approx. 3 celery sticks)
- 2 Tbsp. Extra Virgin Olive Oil (EVOO)
- 2 Tbsp. Green Onion, Chopped
- 2 Tbsp. Dried Parsley
- ½ Tsp. Pure Sea Salt
- ½ Tsp. Garlic Powder
- ⅛ Tsp. Ground Black Pepper

Makes 3-4 servings.

1. Pour the cauliflower into a food processor and blend until it resembles the texture of rice.
2. Heat a large pan to medium and add the EVOO, making sure the oil coats the entire bottom.
3. Add all ingredients and mix until everything is blended, stirring frequently for about 5 minutes.
4. Cover and cook for about 8 minutes or until soft.
5. Serve.

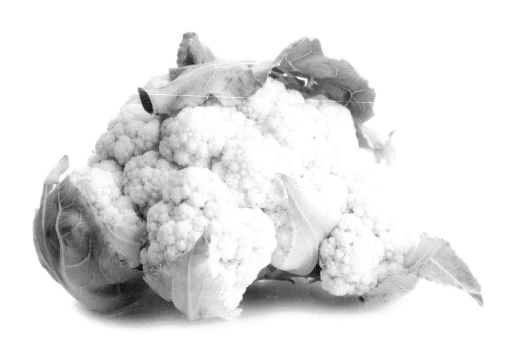

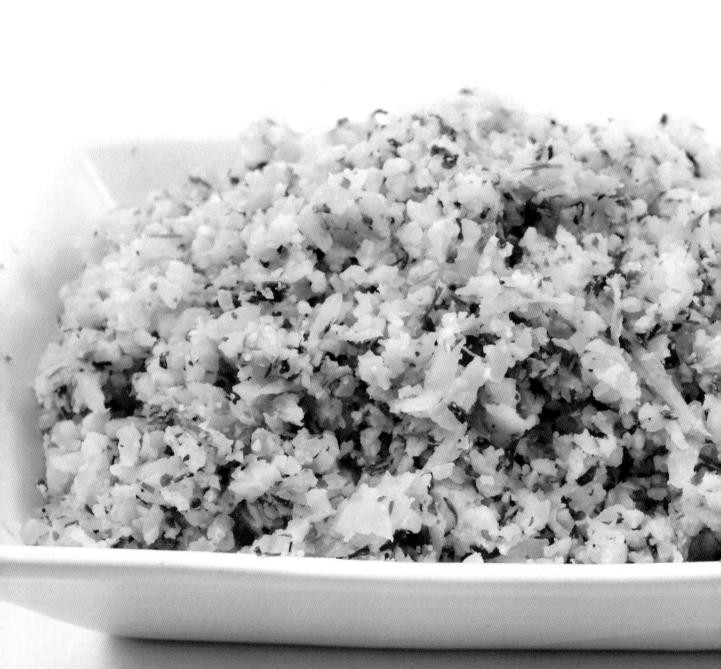

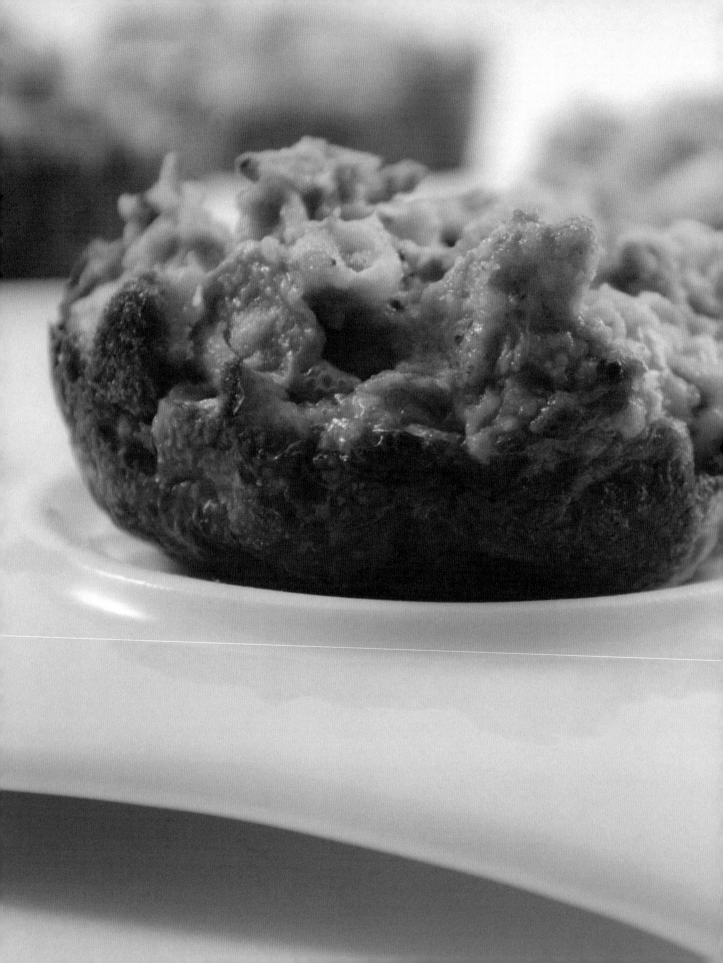

Veggie "Muffins"

This is a great way to "trick" those that may not love veggies. These are not like the zucchini carrot muffins, which are sweet and taste like actual muffins. These are intended to be served as a side item and while they have a touch of sweetness, they are much more salty than sweet. If you cannot eat all 12 muffins within a 4-day period then vacuum seal them and throw them in the freezer for future use!

- 1 Cup Carrots, Finely Chopped
- 1 Cup Celery, Finely Chopped
- 1 Cup Broccoli, Stems Removed and Finely Chopped
- 1 Cup Zucchini, Skin Removed and Finely Chopped
- ½ Cup Onion, Finely Chopped
- ½ Cup Almond Flour, Blanched
- 2 Large Eggs
- 1½ Tbsp. Extra Virgin Olive Oil (EVOO)
- ¼ Tsp. Pure Sea Salt
- ¼ Tsp. Aluminum-Free Baking Soda
- ⅛ Tsp. Ground Black Pepper

Makes 12 veggie "muffins."

1. Preheat the oven to 350 degrees.
2. Spray a large muffin tin with a non-stick spray.
3. Heat a large skillet to medium and then add the EVOO, covering the bottom completely.
4. Add the carrots, celery, onion, and broccoli and sauté for approx. 6 minutes stirring halfway through.
5. Using a large bowl, add the remaining ingredients, and add the cooked carrots, celery, onion, and broccoli. Stir.
6. Using a large spoon, scoop spoonfuls into the muffin tin.
7. Place the muffin tin in the oven on the center rack and bake for 25 minutes.
8. Serve.

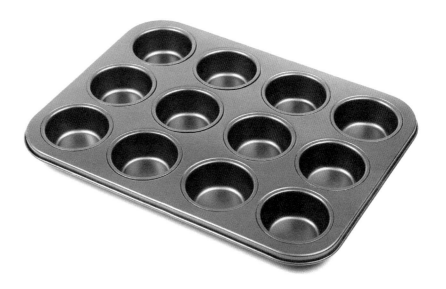

Stuffed Tomatoes

If you are not a fan of tomatoes by themselves (or if you are), you may like this recipe because I've paired the tomatoes with a nice mixture of flavors and textures. This is intended to be served as a side item, but can be eaten alone.

- 4 Large Premium Tomatoes
- ½ Cup Carrots, Finely Chopped
- ½ Cup Mushrooms, Finely Chopped
- ⅓ Cup Celery, Finely Chopped
- ¼ LB Chicken Sausage, Cooked and Minced
- ¼ Cup *Better Breadcrumbs* (page 86)
- 2 Tbsp. Quality Parmesan Cheese
- 1 Tbsp. Extra Virgin Olive Oil (EVOO)
- ½ Tsp. Pure Sea Salt
- ½ Tsp. Garlic Powder
- ¼ Tsp. Onion Powder

Makes 4 stuffed tomatoes.

1. Preheat the oven to 350 degrees.
2. Cover a baking sheet with parchment paper and spray with a non-stick spray.
3. Heat a large skillet to medium and then add the EVOO, covering the bottom completely.
4. Add the carrots, celery, and onion and sauté for approx. 6 minutes stirring halfway through.
5. Cut off the tops of the tomatoes and remove the insides so they resemble a cup.
6. In a large bowl, mix together the remaining ingredients and add the cooked carrots, celery, and onion. Mix.
7. Fill each tomato with the filling and place on the baking sheet.
8. Place the baking sheet in the oven on the center rack and bake for 15-20 minutes.
9. Serve.

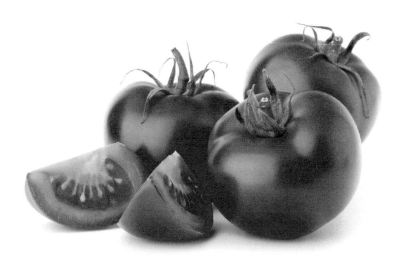

Black Bean Burgers

This is a cost effective way to have "burgers" and provides a good alternative if you do not want meat. After going to Europe in 2012, my eyes were opened up to serving eggs over burgers. Not only do eggs add extra flavor and texture, they add more protein. Make the eggs over easy so they are a bit runny or serve these burgers with *salsa* (page 89).

- 15 oz Can Low-Sodium Black Beans, Drained and Rinsed
- 1 Cup Mushrooms, Finely Chopped
- 2 Large Eggs
- ¼ Cup Quality Parmesan Cheese
- 2 Tbsp. Ground Golden Flaxseed
- 1 Tsp. Cumin
- ½ Tsp. Chili Powder
- ½ Tsp. Pure Sea Salt
- ½ Tsp. Onion Powder
- ½ Tsp. Garlic Powder

Makes 6 burgers.

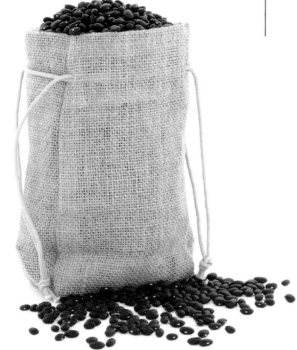

1. Preheat the oven to 375 degrees.
2. Cover a baking sheet with parchment paper and spray with a non-stick spray.
3. Using a food processor, mix together all ingredients until a raw burger like consistency is reached (you may need to stop and use a large spoon to scrap the mixture from the walls of the processor and then continue).
4. Transfer the mixture from the food processor to a large bowl.
5. Form the mixture into large patties and place on the baking sheet about a ½ inch apart.
6. Place the baking sheet in the oven on the center rack and bake for 20 minutes.
7. Remove and flip the burgers over and place the baking sheet back in the oven and bake for an additional 10 minutes.
8. Serve.

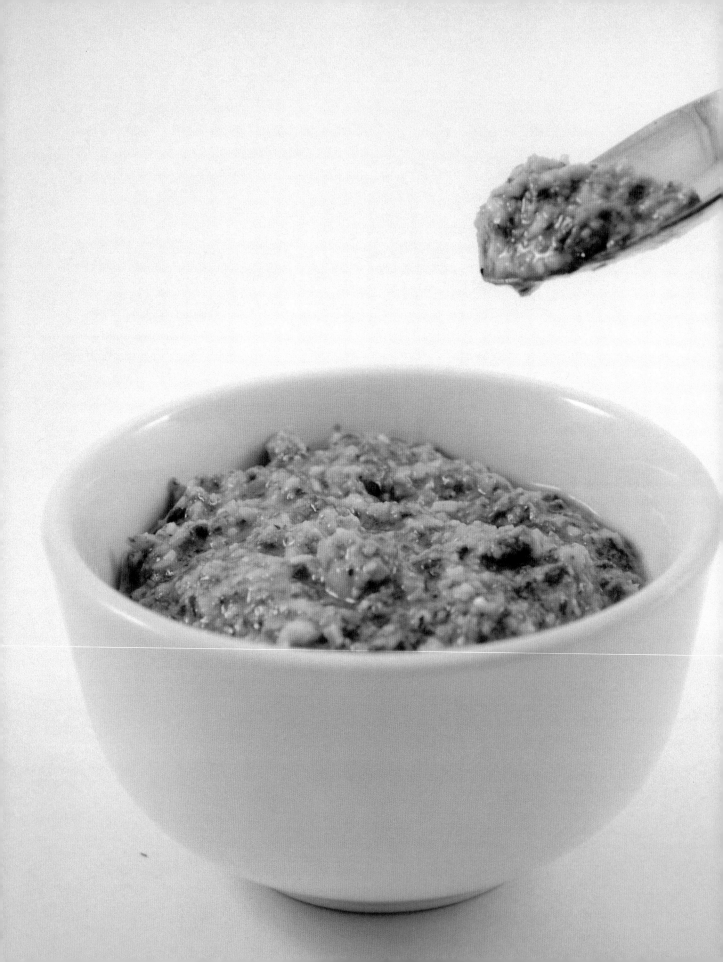

dips, sauces, and seasonings

Better Breadcrumbs

Store bought breadcrumbs are full of unrecognizable ingredients so I make my own. Do I make them every time I need them? No! Who has time for all that? I make a big batch and refrigerate until I need them. Would you believe me if I told you I only have to make breadcrumbs twice a year?

- ½ Package Sprouted Grains Bread, Stale or Toasted
- 1 Tbsp. Dried Thyme
- 1 Tbsp. Dried Parsley
- 1 Tsp. Pure Sea Salt
- ½ Tsp. Garlic Powder
- ¼ Tsp. Ground Black Pepper

Makes approximately 3½ cups.

1. Break the bread into small pieces and add to a food processor (depending on the size of your processor, you may need to do half the bread, remove, and then do the other half).

2. Once all the bread is blended and is fine like breadcrumbs, return the bread back to the processor (if any).

3. Dump in the remaining ingredients and pulse until all seasoning is evenly dispersed.

4. Serve or if you are refrigerating for future use, follow these steps:

   1) Preheat the oven to 300 degrees.

   2) Line a baking sheet with foil and parchment paper-in-one (with the foil face down so it does not touch the breadcrumbs).

   3) Pour all breadcrumbs onto the baking sheet.

   4) Place on the center rack and bake for 15 minutes or until golden brown.

   5) Remove and place in a sealed container in the refrigerator for up to 6 months.

tip

Instead of using a new package of bread, save your leftover bread scraps (from cutting bread thinner and from the *vegged-out "egg-in-the-middle"* (page 42) and place in sandwich bags in the refrigerator. Once you have approximately 8 bags full of scraps, you are ready to make another batch!

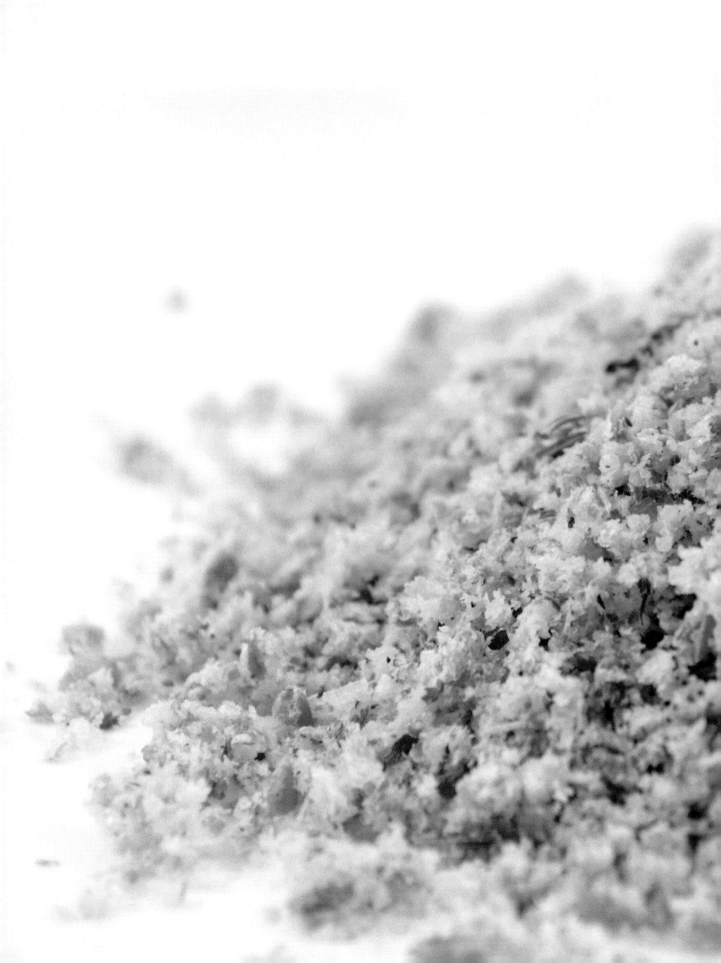

Guacamole

My dad loved fresh ingredients so this reminds me of him. It is super easy and bursts with flavor. Cilantro and citrus just work so well together. Do you like your guacamole spicy? Just add some jalapeno or more red pepper flakes.

- 1 Hass Avocado, Pitted
- 2 Tbsp. Tomato, Chopped
- 2 Tsp. Red Onion, Chopped
- 1 Tsp. Fresh Cilantro, Chopped
- ¼ Tsp. Pure Sea Salt
- ¼ Tsp. Red Pepper Flakes
- 2 Big Squeezes of Half a Lime

Makes 2 servings.

1. Scoop the bright green meat out of the avocado, place in a medium sized bowl, and then discard the shell.
2. Add the remaining ingredients.
3. Mash with a fork until the mixture is a creamy texture.
4. Serve.

tip

This will last about 2 days in the refrigerator. Avocado meat loses its bright green coloring when refrigerated, but mixing it with a spoon will bring it back.

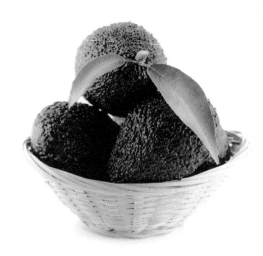

Salsa

I will always have memories of my dad chopping fresh vegetables and herbs in the kitchen. I think he was happiest in these moments and with the amazing aromas that come from fresh herbs, I can see why! After you see how simple homemade salsa can be, I bet you will never buy it pre made again! If you like your salsa spicy, just add in a jalapeno or more red pepper flakes.

- 1 Cup Tomatoes, Chopped
- 1 Small Lime, Squeezed
- 2 Tbsp. Red Onion, Chopped
- 1 Tbsp. Fresh Cilantro, Chopped
- ¼ Tsp. Pure Sea Salt
- ¼ Tsp. Red Pepper Flakes
- ⅛ Tsp. Garlic, Minced

Makes 2 servings.

1. Mix together all ingredients and mash with a fork until the consistency is a chunky liquid.
2. Serve.

tip

Invest in a jar of organic pre chopped garlic. It will save you time and that sticky feeling you get from fresh garlic cloves. The organic jars are found in the refrigerated produce section.

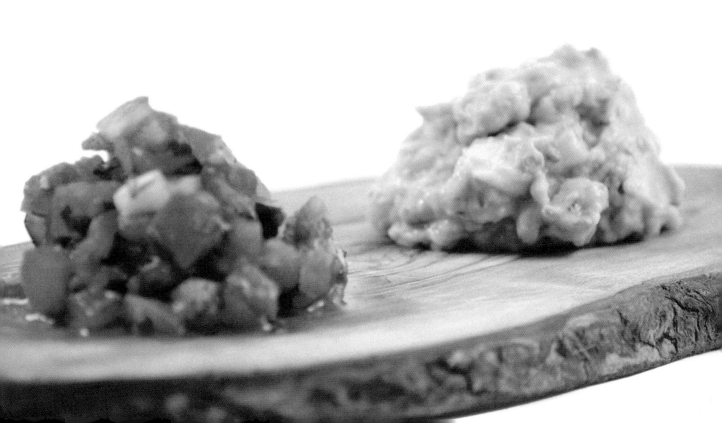

Dry Rub (or Not) Seasoning

Dry rub seasoning is so versatile – you can rub or just use a shake/sprinkle method. You can dry rub chicken breasts and marinate in the refrigerator, you can rub a turkey and cook in a slow cooker. You can add to fish, potatoes, and more! It has a great color and lasts for up to 6 months in the refrigerator!

- ¼ Cup Paprika
- 3 Tbsp. Pure Sea Salt
- 3 Tbsp. Garlic Powder
- 2½ Tbsp. Ground Black Pepper
- 1½ Tbsp. Onion Powder
- 1¼ Tbsp. Dried Oregano
- 1¼ Tbsp. Dried Thyme
- 1 Tbsp. Chili Pepper

Makes approximately 1 cup.

1. Using a bowl, add all ingredients together and stir with a fork.
2. Place in a sealed container in the refrigerator and store for up to 6 months.

French Onion Dip

French onion dip is typically made with sour cream and a packet full of pre made spices (and other ingredients) that you dump into the sour cream, mix, and serve. Have you ever looked at the list of ingredients included in these packages? I have, and that is why I created my own version! Plain Greek yogurt is a great alternative to sour cream because it is high in protein and the consistency and taste are so similar.

- ¾ Cup Plain Greek Yogurt
- ½ Cup Onions, Cut in Strips
- 1 Tbsp. Extra Virgin Olive Oil (EVOO)
- ½ Tsp. Onion Powder
- ¼ Tsp. Pure Sea Salt
- ¼ Tsp. Organic Worcestershire Sauce
- ⅛ Tsp. Ground Pepper
- ⅛ Tsp. Garlic Powder

Makes 3-4 servings.

1. Heat a small pan to medium and then add the EVOO so that it coats the pan evenly.
2. Add the onions, a small pinch of salt, and then sauté for about 5-7 minutes, mixing frequently with a spatula.
3. Once the onions are caramelized, remove, and set aside.
4. With the exception of the onions, mix together the remaining ingredients in a medium sized bowl.
5. Once the onions have cooled off, add to the dip and mix with a spoon.
6. Serve as a dip for your favorite veggies.

Basil Zucchini Pesto

Basil is one of my favorite fresh herbs because the aroma is so distinct! This is a bit different from traditional pesto recipes because I add zucchini to it. This is great as a "sauce" for *zucchini noodles* (page 39) mixed with shrimp and cherry tomatoes, as a topping on baked chicken, or even as a spread.

- 1 Cup Fresh Basil Leaves, Packed
- ½ Cup Chopped Zucchini, Skins Removed
- ¼ Cup Extra Virgin Olive Oil
- ¼ Cup Parmesan Cheese
- 3 Tbsp. Pine Nuts
- ½ Tsp. Fresh Garlic
- ¼ Tsp. Pure Sea Salt
- ⅛ Tsp. Ground Black Pepper

Makes approximately 1 cup.

1. Using a food processor, add all ingredients and pulse.
2. Stop and scrap the sides of the processor and then continue pulsing until you achieve a dip consistency.
3. Serve.

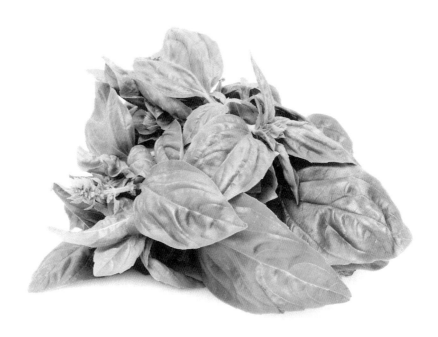

Balsamic Vinaigrette

There are so many options for homemade salad dressings. With a salad shaker (shown), it makes coming up with fresh dressings as easy as adding ingredients and then shaking to perfection!

- 1 Tbsp. + 1 Tsp. Extra Virgin Olive Oil
- ½ Tbsp. Balsamic Vinegar
- 1 Pinch Pure Sea Salt
- ½ Pinch Ground Black Pepper
- 1 Big Squeeze ½ Lime (or a Lemon)
- ⅛ Tsp. Raw Honey

Makes 2 servings.

1. Using a salad shaker, add all ingredients, and shake, shake, shake!
2. Serve.

Healthy Ranch Dressing

- ¼ Cup Plain Greek Yogurt
- 1 Tbsp. 1% Milk
- ½ Tsp. Lemon, Freshly Squeezed
- ¼ Tsp. Dried Parsley
- ⅛ Tsp. Pure Sea Salt
- ⅛ Tsp. Garlic Powder
- ⅛ Tsp. Onion Powder
- ⅛ Tsp. Dried Dill
- Pepper to Taste

Makes 2 servings.

1. Add all ingredients to a medium sized bowl and mix with a fork.
2. Serve.

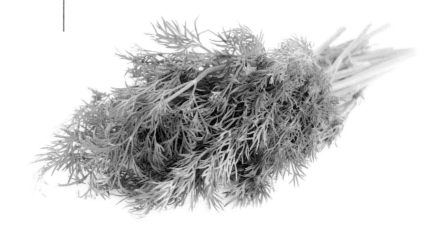

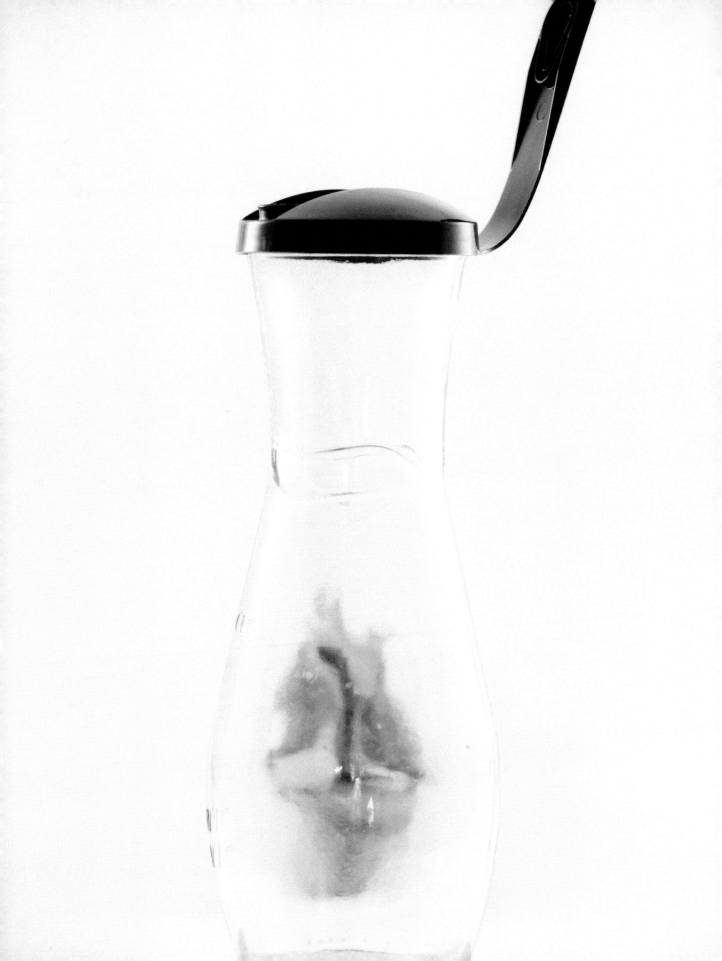

Fajitas Seasoning

Have you tried finding a fajitas seasoning packet that has recognizable ingredients?
It is hard to find so here's a simple recipe you can whip up!

- ½ Cup Water
- 2½ Tsp. Chili Powder
- 1 Tsp. Organic Cornstarch
- 1 Tsp. Pure Sea Salt
- 1 Tsp. Paprika
- 1 Tsp. Raw Coconut Sugar
  (Granulated Powder)
- ½ Tsp. Cumin
- ¼ Tsp. Garlic Powder
- ¼ Tsp. Onion Powder
- ¼ Tsp. Pure Unsweetened Cocoa
- ¼ Tsp. Dried Oregano

Makes 4 servings.

1. Combine all ingredients in a measuring cup and mix with a fork until all clumps are gone.
2. Heat a medium sized pan to medium and then pour the fajitas liquid into the pan.
3. Stir frequently until the liquid is hot and starts to thicken.
4. Pour over cooked chicken, rice, onions, and peppers and serve with lettuce, tomatoes, and Greek yogurt.

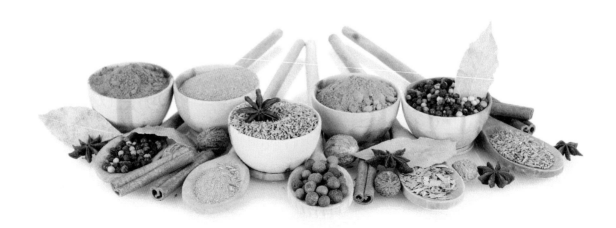

Brown Gravy

Brown gravy packets are convenient, but they are full of sodium and unrecognizable ingredients. There is an alternative! I use this in my *cauliflower shepherd's "pie"* (page 65).

- 1 Cup Organic Beef Broth
- 1 Tbsp. Salted Butter
- 1 Tbsp. Organic Cornstarch
- 1 Tsp. Pure Sea Salt
- ½ Tsp. Garlic Powder
- ¼ Tsp. Onion Powder
- ⅛ Tsp. Ground Black Pepper

Makes 4 servings.

1. Heat a large pan to medium and add the butter, making sure it evenly coats the bottom of the pan.
2. In a bowl, mix together the broth and the cornstarch with a fork.
3. Once all clumps are gone, pour in the remaining ingredients and mix.
4. Pour all the liquid in the pan and stir continuously until it thickens.
5. Serve.

Simple Chicken Marinade

Marinating chicken in the refrigerator is a guarantee that you will have a moist and tasty result. Here's a very simple one using just a few ingredients.

- ⅓ Cup Extra Virgin Olive Oil
- 2 Tbsp. Raw Honey
- 1 Med. Lemon, Fully Squeezed
- ½ Tsp. Pure Sea Salt

Makes 4 servings.

1. Using a fork, mix all ingredients in a bowl.
2. Add approximately 1 lb. of raw chicken breasts to a plastic storage bag.
3. Pour the marinade into the bag, close, and massage from the outside so that all breasts are evenly coated with the marinade.
4. Place in the refrigerator overnight (12 hours) or for a minimum of 3 hours.
5. Once ready, cook the chicken as you would normally.

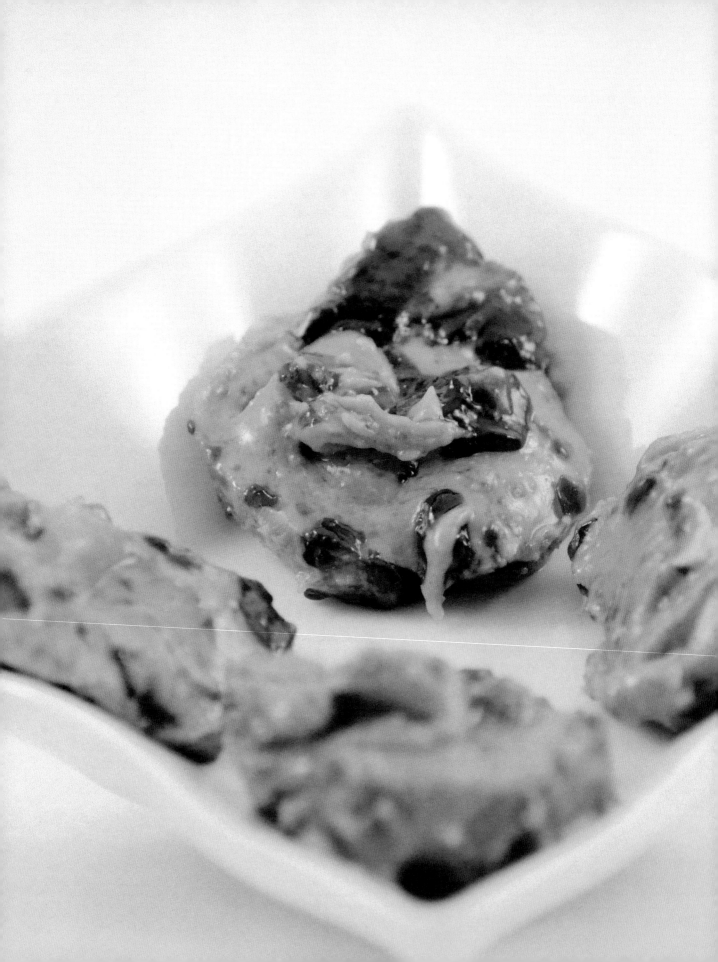

desserts

Healthier Chocolate Chip "Cookies"

Chocolate chip cookies are by far our favorite dessert. By using almond flour, golden flaxseed, applesauce, and coconut nectar, these are a much healthier alternative to traditional cookie recipes. For those of you that like your cookies soft then this is the recipe for you! Just try not to eat the entire batch!

Dry Ingredients:

- 1½ Cup Almond Flour, Blanched
- ½ Cup Ground Golden Flaxseed
- ½ Tsp. Pure Sea Salt
- ¼ Tsp. Aluminum-Free Baking Soda

Wet Ingredients:

- 2 Large Eggs
- ¼ Cup Grapeseed Oil
- ⅓ Cup + 2 Tbsp. Coconut Nectar
- 2 Tbsp. Unsweetened Applesauce
- 1 Tbsp. Pure Vanilla Extract
- ½ Cup Chocolate Chips, Semi-Sweet

Makes approximately 18 cookies.

1. Preheat the oven to 350 degrees.
2. Cover 2 baking sheets with parchment paper and spray with a non-stick spray or rub with coconut oil.
3. Using a large bowl, mix together all the dry ingredients.
4. Using a large bowl (preferably with a handle and a spout), mix together all the wet ingredients with the exception of the chocolate chips.
5. Pour the dry ingredients into the wet ingredients.
6. Stir with a large spoon until the batter is free of clumps.
7. Add the chocolate chips and fold them into the batter.
8. Using a small spoon, scoop spoonfuls of the cookie mixture onto the baking sheets, leaving 2 inches between each cookie.
9. Place on the center rack and bake for 18 minutes.
10. Remove and let cool for a minimum of 15 minutes to firm up.
11. Serve.

tip

Want even healthier chocolate chip cookies? Add ⅓ cup of chopped zucchini and replace the semi-sweet chocolate with dark chocolate.

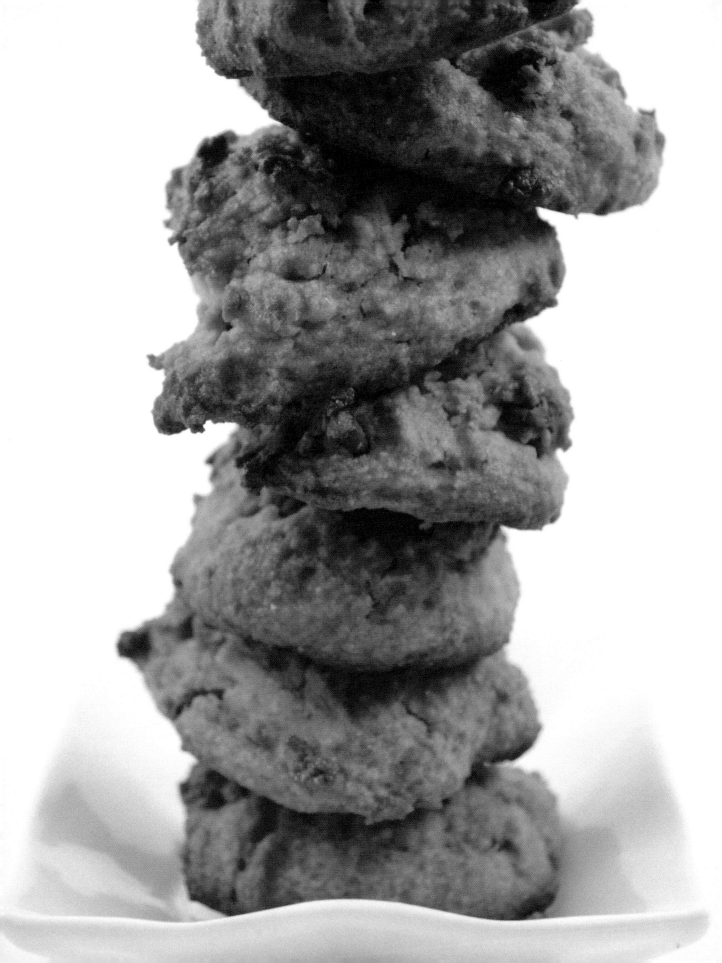

Almond Date Sheets

If you are looking for something that melts in your mouth then this is the recipe! These are high in protein and use chopped dates, which are very sweet and have a nice texture when baked. If you are looking for more texture then add chopped walnuts or pecans.

Dry Ingredients:

- 1 Cup Almond Flour, Blanched
- 1 Scoop Quality Vanilla Protein Powder (approx. 1.5 oz.)
- ¼ Tsp. Pure Sea Salt
- ¼ Tsp. Aluminum-Free Baking Soda

Wet Ingredients:

- 2 Large Eggs
- ¼ Cup Raw Coconut Nectar
- ¼ Cup Grapeseed Oil
- 2 Tbsp. Unsweetened Applesauce
- 1 Tbsp. Pure Vanilla Extract
- 1 Cup Chopped Dates, Pitted (approx. 15)

Makes 10 servings.

1. Preheat the oven to 350 degrees.
2. Cover a baking sheet with parchment paper and lightly spray with a non-stick spray or rub with coconut oil.
3. Using a large bowl, mix together all dry ingredients with a fork.
4. Using a large bowl (preferably with a handle and a spout), mix together all the wet ingredients with the exception of the dates.
5. Pour the dry ingredients into the wet ingredients.
6. Stir with a large spoon until the mixture is free of clumps (the mixture will be thin).
7. Add the chopped dates and fold into the mixture.
8. Pour the mixture onto the baking sheet.
9. Place on the center rack and bake for 15-20 minutes or until golden brown.
10. Serve.

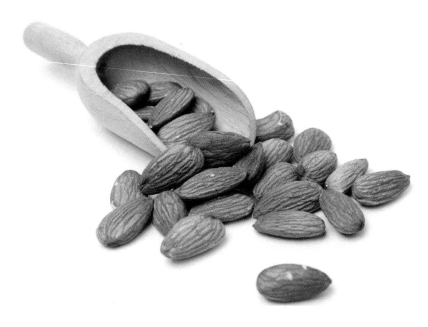

Chocolate Protein Frozen "Candy"

I love playing around with texture of food. By placing this in the freezer, it gives it a candy like consistency.

- 1 Scoop Quality Chocolate Protein Powder (approx. 1.5 oz.)
- ¼ Cup Sunbutter, Creamy or Crunchy
- 2 Tbsp. Unsweetened Almond Milk
- ½ Tsp. Ground Golden Flaxseed
- ½ Tsp. Pure Vanilla Extract

Makes 8 "candy" pieces.

1. Using a medium bowl, mix together all ingredients with a spoon.
2. Using a small spoon, scoop the mixture into a mini muffin tin.
3. Cover with foil and parchment paper-in-one (with the parchment side touching the food) and place in the freezer for a minimum of 3 hours.
4. Serve.

tip

Do not leave these out for long as they melt quickly and become messy.

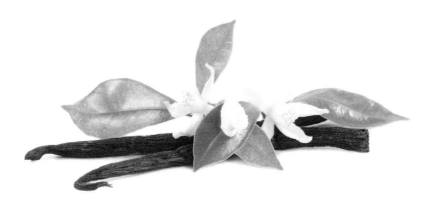

PB&J Frozen "Candy"

My husband is not a huge fan of peanut butter and jelly (PB&J), but I think he may be the only person that feels this way. I absolutely love PB&J and had to find a way to get my dose of it without slathering it on two pieces of bread. Knowing that PB firms up in the freezer, I started experimenting. What I ended up with is an extremely simple recipe that has satisfied my PB&J urge many nights!

- ¼ Cup Unsweetened Organic Peanut Butter, Creamy
- ¼ Cup Grape Jelly

Makes 10 "candy" pieces.

1. Using a small bowl, add the PB and then fold in the jelly.
2. Using a small spoon, scoop the mixture into a mini muffin tin.
3. Cover with foil and parchment paper-in-one, (with the parchment side facing the food) and place in the freezer for a minimum of 3 hours.
4. Serve.

tip

It is important that you do not stir excessively as you want there to be chunks of jelly within each of the candy pieces. For this reason, I do not recommend using jam or spread since they are too runny and do not yield the same result.

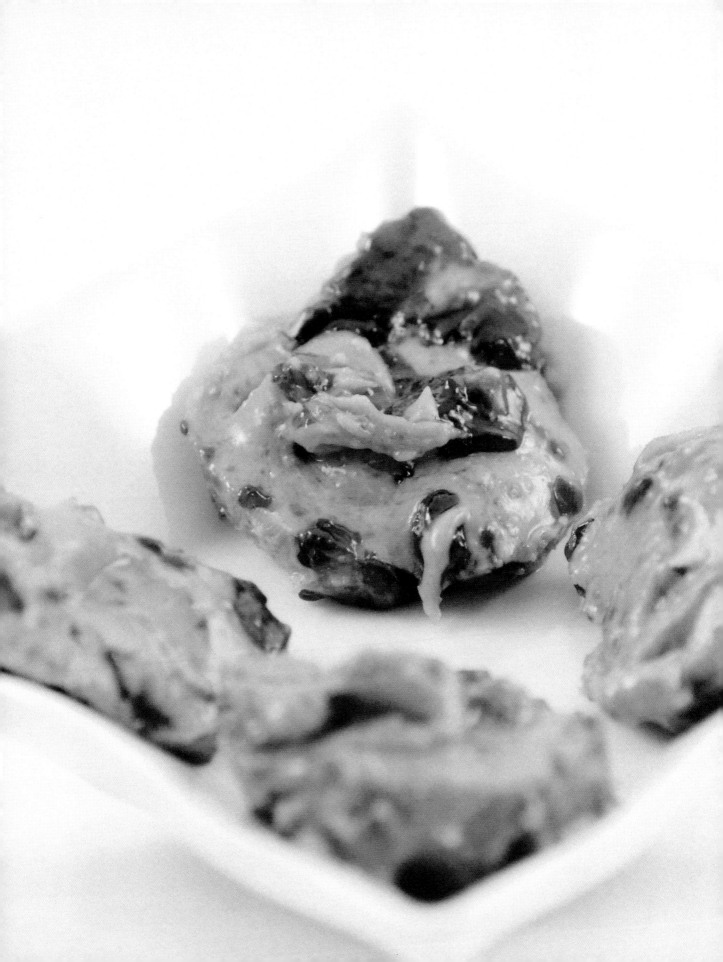

Common Desserts Using Fruit

Banana with Peanut Butter

Do you like the banana and peanut butter combination? If so, you must try a frozen version! The PB becomes firm making it a great texture and the banana stays soft while providing the sweetness.

1. Peel a very ripe banana, cut in half, and then again so you end up with 4 equal cuts.

2. Spread organic unsweetened PB, unsweetened almond butter, or sunbutter on 2 of the banana cuts.

3. Take 2 sticks (or coffee stirs) and place towards the bottom of each of the banana cuts that have PB on them.

4. Take the 2 banana cuts that do not have PB on them and put on top of the banana cuts with the PB.

5. Cover both bananas with foil and parchment paper-in-one (with the parchment side touching the food) and freeze for a minimum of 4 hours.

6. Serve.

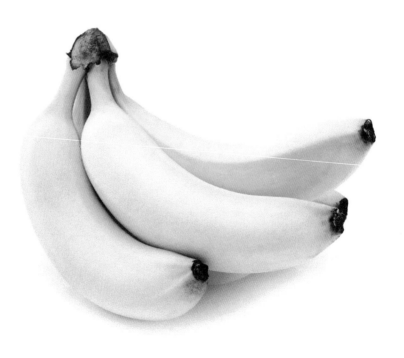

Common Desserts Using Fruit

Chocolate Covered Fruit

When I learned how easy it is to make chocolate covered fruit, I rarely ever buy it. Not only is it less expensive, the chocolate firms up super quick making an almost instant treat!

1. Clean your fruit of choice. I like strawberries but any will do.
2. If you are using strawberries, cut the leaves off.
3. Melt approximately ¼ cup of dark chocolate by placing in the microwave for 30 seconds. Stir. If necessary, melt for an additional 30 seconds, but watch carefully because you do not want burnt chocolate.
4. Alternatively, you can melt the chocolate by placing it in a small glass bowl over a slightly bigger pot over low heat. Make sure to constantly stir to reduce the chance of the chocolate burning.
5. Once the chocolate is melted, start dipping your fruit, place on a paper plate, and put in the refrigerator. It will take approximately 30 minutes for the chocolate to become hard and it will lift right off the plate.
6. Serve.

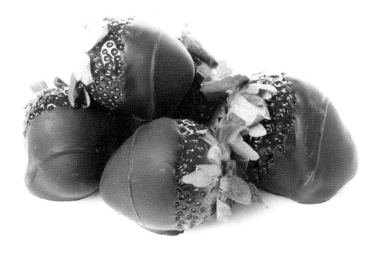

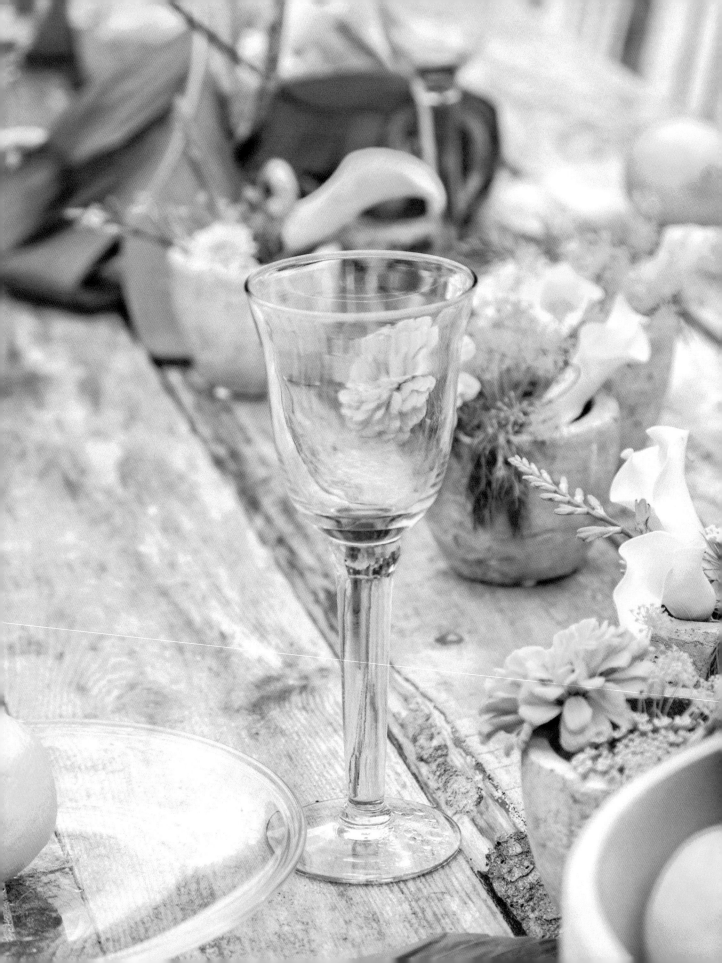

party menu

Party Menu

When you think of party menus, you likely do not classify them as being healthy. There are many options that you can add to your menu that are healthier for you, are simple to make, and are crowd pleasers. In addition to the recipes below, here are some other options for you:

1. Serve up *turkey zucchini meatballs* (page 61) in a slow cooker.

2. Serve up *salsa* (page 89), *guacamole* (page 88), *french onion dip* (page 90), or *healthy ranch dressing* (page 92) with vegetables and/or organic baked chips made of seeds and sprouted grains.

3. Offer lettuce wraps as an option for guests that may not want bread.

4. Offer a mixed salad with a combination of greens, colorful vegetables, seeds and nuts, and raisins.

5. Pair the salad with *balsamic vinaigrette* (page 92) and *healthy ranch dressing* (page 92).

6. Make muffins (page 49, 50, and 51) as mini muffins.

7. Serve *healthier chocolate chip "cookies"* (page 98), *almond date sheets* (page 100), or *chocolate covered fruit* (page 105).

Deviled Eggs Filled with Guacamole

Egg whites + guacamole = a nutritional powerhouse. This is a unique way to bring together two of the most common party favorites—deviled eggs and guacamole dip. You can also combine other favorites, such as eggs with tuna or chicken salad.

• 10 Large Eggs, *Hard Boiled* (page 36)

• 2 Servings *Guacamole* (page 88)

Makes 20 guacamole filled eggs.

1. Cut the eggs in half lengthwise.

2. Remove the yolks.

3. Place all the eggs on a big plate or on an egg platter.

4. Scoop small spoonfuls of guacamole into each of the egg holes.

5. Cover with plastic and place in the refrigerator.

6. Serve.

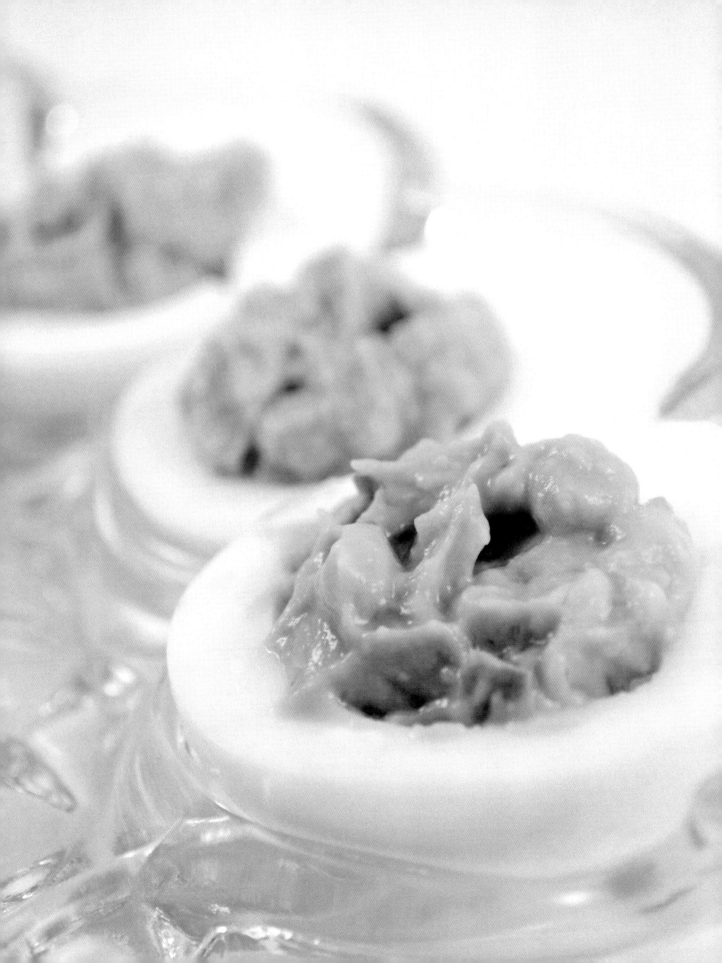

Chicken Apple Sausage on a Stick

This is probably the easiest of all menu items. You can pre cook the chicken sausage or just buy it pre cooked. The sausage and apple combination gives a nice salty and sweet result and it is great served cold.

- 1 LB Chicken Sausage, Cooked
- 2 Apples

Makes approximately 30 chicken apple sausage appetizers.

1. Cut the chicken sausage into ½ inch-thick rounds.
2. Cut the apples into ½ inch-thick chunks.
3. Using toothpicks, layer a chicken sausage round and then an apple chunk. Repeat with approx. 30 toothpicks.
4. Serve.

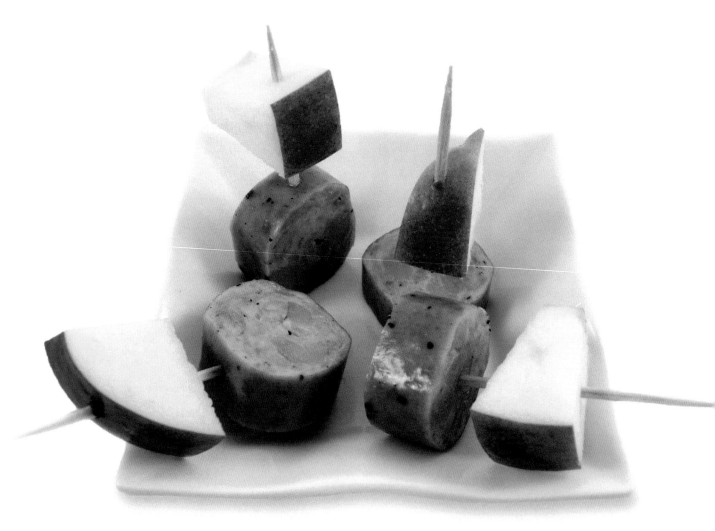

Turkey-Bacon-Wrapped Dates on a Stick

This is one of my favorites. I actually have to stop myself from eating these because they are the perfect combination of salty and sweet and are easy to eat!

• 8 oz. Package Turkey Bacon, No Nitrates or Nitrites Added

• 24 Dates, Pitted

Makes 24 turkey-bacon-wrapped appetizers.

1. Preheat the oven to 400 degrees.

2. Cover a baking sheet with parchment paper and lightly spray with a non-stick spray.

3. Cut each bacon strip in 3 pieces so that you end up with 24 pieces total.

4. Take a date and wrap each with a turkey bacon strip and stick it with a toothpick to hold it together. Repeat.

5. Place the baking sheet on the center rack and bake for 20-25 minutes or until the bacon is no longer pink.

6. Serve.

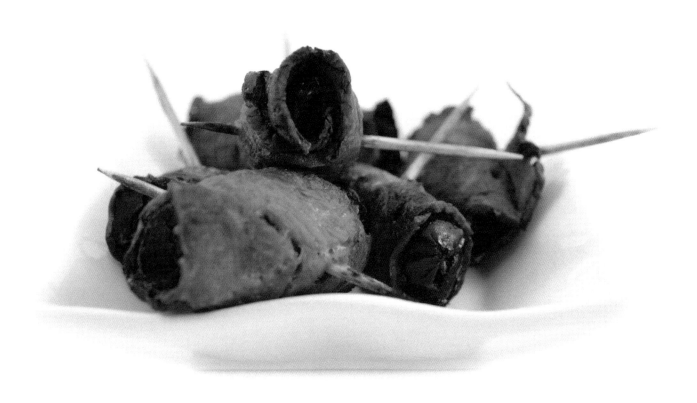

Crunchy Fruit Salad

This is my mother-in-law's recipe and every time she makes it, I devour it. I made only 1 change. Instead of using mayonnaise, I use Greek yogurt.

- 2 Apples, Cut in Chunks (approx. 3½ Cups)
- 1 Cup Pineapple, Cut in Small Pieces
- 1 Cup Grapes, Cut in Half
- ½ Cup Raisins
- ½ Cup Pecans or Walnuts
- ½ Cup Plain Greek Yogurt
- ¼ Cup Celery, Chopped
- ½ Tsp. Pure Sea Salt

Makes approximately 6 cups.

1. Combine all ingredients together.
2. Serve.

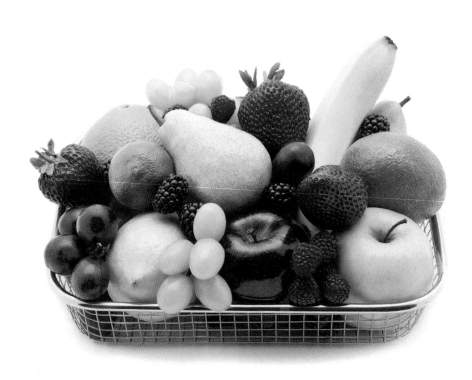

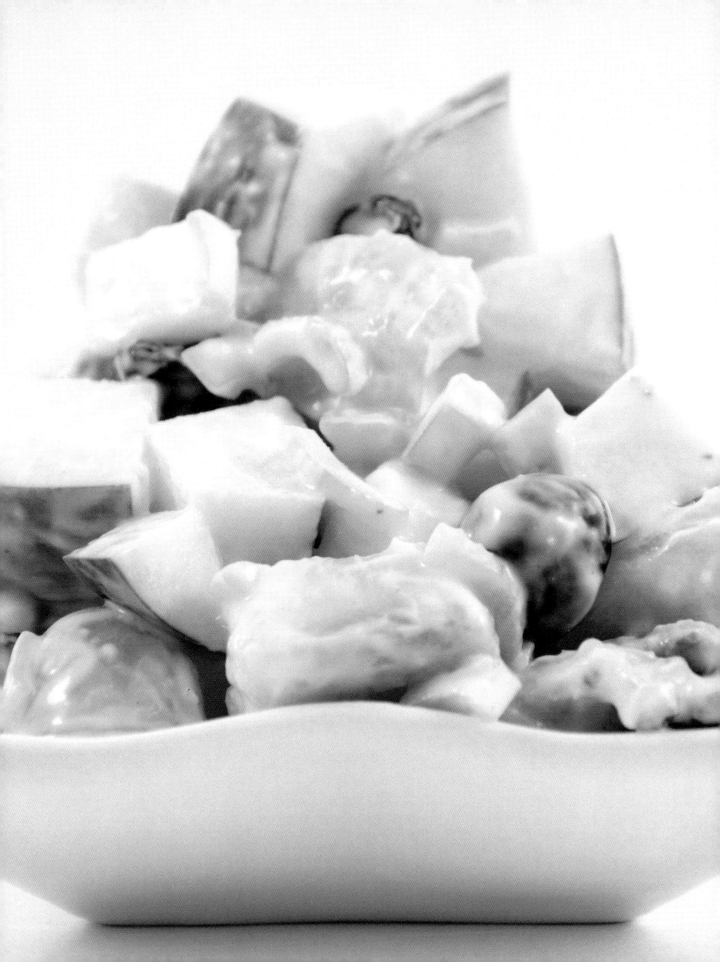

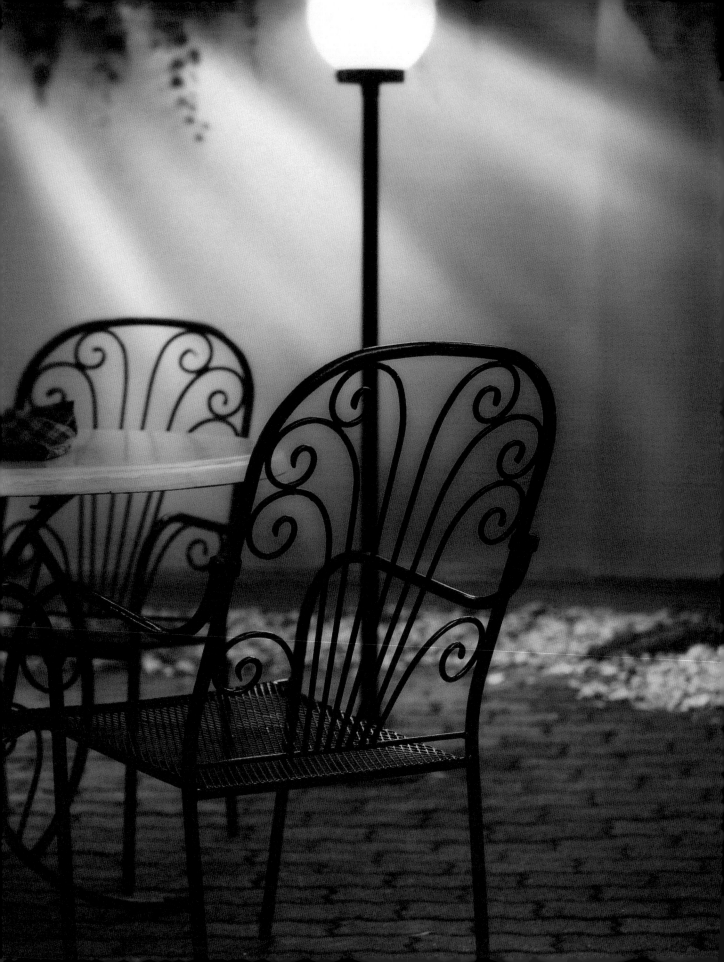

dining out
and traveling

Many people believe that if you are eating healthy, then you cannot go out to eat. This is simply not true. Remember, this is not a diet; it is a way of life. With a little education and preparation, you will see that there are a lot of options, especially with the growing health-minded companies that want to offer healthier options to the consumer.

First, if you have eaten healthy and worked out all week long, then a cheat meal may not be a bad choice for you. So, go out and enjoy what you have earned. When you start to make that one meal turn into days of cheat meals, then you are going to start feeling it.

Do you just want a good healthy option when you go out? Here's what you want to look for:

1. Restaurants that take pride in the quality of their food, including how the animals are raised for the meats they prepare, how produce and grains are grown (without the use of pesticides), and how the company deals with impacts to the environment (using recyclable material, etc.). Typically these companies offer healthy options.

2. Restaurants that change their menu based on what is in season. These venues typically cook with fresh ingredients.

3. Restaurants that use fish they catch from the sea and serve the same day. They will likely have a lot of fresh seafood options.

4. Restaurants that do not use MSG or other unhealthy preservatives and additives in their food.

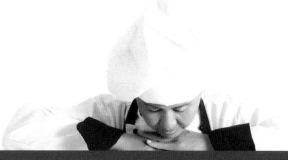

Have you gotten to "that place" we spoke about at the beginning of the book? Don't panic! If you are forced to stop to eat somewhere out of convenience and desperation, just make sure you order a protein (chicken, fish, turkey), ask for it to be grilled, and include a side of fruits and vegetables if available.

Once you have done your research and found a viable place at which to dine, here are some of the healthier options:

1. Elect grilled or baked fish and eliminate any cream sauces.
2. Instead of a loaded baked potato, ask for a sweet potato with cinnamon and real butter on the side.
3. For salads, try to get freshly made vinaigrette dressings instead of creamy options.
4. Always ask for a protein, such as fish or chicken, to be added.
5. Ordering an organic beef burger or a veggie burger? Ask the server to bring it "open faced," which means it only has the bottom part of the bun. Using a knife and fork will actually be less messy, and it will probably take you longer to eat it.
6. Order a broth-based soup as your appetizer in lieu of munching on breads and tortilla chips.

Now you know how to dine out, so you can apply this when you are traveling. Part of traveling to other areas and learning about a given culture is through their food. So, try to balance healthiness without compromising true enjoyment of a specific region's culture.

When I travel, especially for work, I don't find it difficult to find healthy options when I go to a restaurant to eat breakfast, lunch, or dinner; it is the traveling back and forth part and snacking that are challenging. So, what do I do? I prepare myself!

Before any work trip, not only do I make food for my husband for when I am gone (yes, I know I'm a good wife!), I also prepare food that I can bring on the plane with me. This includes making baked turkey bacon and high-protein muffins, as well as bringing raw nuts/ seeds and fruits that do not need refrigeration, such as apples, bananas, and oranges. I make sure to have a well-balanced meal before leaving for the airport, so my snacks should hold me over until more options are available to me.

For a weeklong work trip, these snacks will last me about three or four days, which means I need to go buy food for my travel-back day. Most cities have a grocery store that is within a reasonable distance, so I just go the night before traveling and pick up the essentials. I eat a well-balanced meal before going to the airport, and I am all set.

I get a lot of questions about how to eat while on a cruise. We all know cruises give us essentially 24/7 access to food. Would you believe me if I told you I once lost weight while on a cruise (and no, I was not sick!)? While no one expects you to lose weight while cruising, here are some suggestions so you feel good at the end of the trip:

1. Just because dessert is offered for breakfast, lunch, and dinner does not mean you should eat it. In our household, we typically only eat dessert on the weekend, so it is easy for us to indulge in dessert only a few nights on the cruise. At a minimum, try to reserve dessert for after dinner.

2. Bread is an easy food to mindlessly chomp on (and we know the bread is good on cruises). Treat bread like a dessert and limit how much you eat. Frankly, with the option to order everything on the menu, I would rather try a new soup or fish then fill up on bread.

3. Treat pancakes, waffles, French toast, and bagels like you would dessert. While you can have them, don't make it a habit every day. Instead, stick to options like eggs, oatmeal, and fruits. You will feel better in the long run.

4. Bring nuts and seeds to snack on.

5. Ditch the elevators. Instead, use the stairs throughout the cruise and burn calories.

6. Take advantage of the health and fitness facilities and classes on board. When are you able to run laps out in the middle of the ocean? Or work out in a gym that overlooks the sunset? Most people do not use the fitness facilities, so you can always get a machine!

7. Most importantly, be reasonable. If you are not eating something at home, then think twice about eating it on the cruise. If you feel you deserve it, then go for it!

> **tip**
>
> When in doubt, just ask the server if the food is made with MSG or other additives. You can also ask for alternative menus, such as gluten free and vegetarian.

If you have learned anything from this book, I hope it is to have purpose behind your eating decisions and be as prepared as you possibly can. Living a healthy lifestyle can be done. People all over the world have demanding lives and figure out how to do it. You can, too. Take the tips and strategies that I have laid out and figure out what works for you. It is all about trying different techniques until you finally figure out your own way.

Menu

AMA
Restaurant

ς ήρθατε

Bienvenu

venuti

notes

Environmental Working Group—"Dirty Dozen" and "Clean Fifteen" Organic Guide
Copyright © Environmental Working Group, www.ewg.org
Reprinted with permission.

Medline Plus (US National Library of Medicine and National Institutes of Health)—Antioxidants
http://www.nlm.nih.gov/medlineplus/antioxidants.html

United States Department of Agriculture (USDA)—Definitions: Organic, Grass Fed; Inflammation; National Nutrient Database; Farmers Market Database
www.usda.gov

USDA—Food Standards & Labeling Policy Book
http://www.fsis.usda.gov/OPPDE/larc/Policies/Labeling_Policy_Book_082005.pdf

United States Food and Drug Administration (FDA)—Common Food Allergens; Food Labeling; Food Storage
www.fda.gov

University of Sydney, Home of the Glycemic Index—Definition; Glycemic Rankings
www.glycemicindex.com

index

index

index

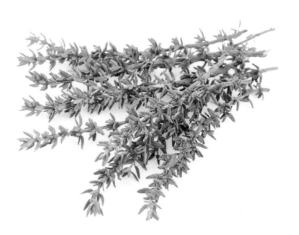